I0791156

ISBN: 9781678483265

30-DAY Gluten Free No-Cooking Diet

Gail Johnson, M. S.
Ron Hill, Jr.

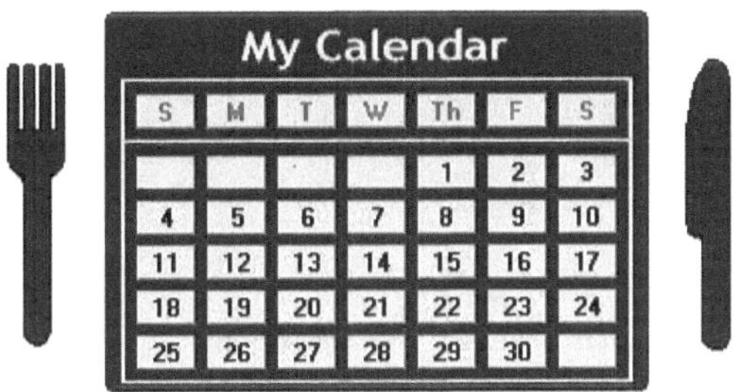

NoPaperPress™

Note: At publication, the off-the-shelf foods used in this book were widely available in most supermarkets. But food products come and go. So if there is a frozen entrée or soup selection in this diet that is out of stock, or that's been discontinued, or perhaps you don't like, or that you forgot to pick up while shopping, please substitute another food that has **approximately** the same caloric value and nutritional content. In this regard, many dieters have found the foods listed in the Appendices at the end of this book to be very helpful.

CONTENTS

Most of us are busy – extremely busy struggling to balance career, family, finances, and then you need to make room for a personal life, for friends, for learning, for travel and the list goes on and on. Because you're so busy, you may neglect your health. You know you should lose weight. You want to lose weight but don't have the time to diet! Your life is just too hectic to plan and prepare elaborate low-calorie meals. That's where the *30-Day Gluten Free No-Cooking Diet* can help.

According to the late Dr. Jean Mayer of Tufts University's Department of Nutrition, a really good weight-loss diet must have the following three characteristics:

1) The diet must provide you with an understanding of weight control as well as the knowledge you need to reduce your weight to the desired level.
2) The diet must help you remain healthy while you are losing weight.
3) The diet must lead you to a healthier way of eating and exercising that will, in the long term, help you keep off the weight you have lost.

The weight-loss diet featured in this eBook is a so-called "balanced diet;" i.e., a diet that is not only low calorie and reasonably low in fat, but is also nutritionally balanced. The *30-Day Gluten Free No-Cooking Diet*, however, does not meet all the criteria set forth above. While you will get some "dieting insight" and some idea of how much you can eat and still lose weight, you will not get a real understanding of weight control from this eBook. That's not its purpose. What you will get is a healthy diet – and a diet that if followed will promote weight loss – but it's not the long-term answer.

Long-term success is about developing both an understanding and a plan that will result in healthier eating and physical activity habits. The desire to lose weight and the discipline to start and stay on a weight-control program are crucial. But along with desire and discipline, it is our belief that **only an in-depth understanding of weight control, nutrition and exercise will lead to long-term success**. For a through understanding and the guidance you need to succeed in the long term we recommend you read, *Weight Control - U.S. Edition* by Vincent Antonetti, Ph.D., an eBook also published by NoPaperPress.

Before you begin any weight loss program you need to make sure your health will allow you to lower your caloric intake and increase your physical activity. A **medical checkup** is in order which may be as simple as a visit to a physician who is familiar with your medical history, or it may be a thorough physical exam. The physician conducting the medical exam should be made aware of and should approve the specific weight loss diet you're planning   In particular, you should **let your physician know that the 30-Day Gluten Free No-Cooking Diet relies to a considerable degree on**

commercially processed frozen foods – most of which have a relatively high salt (sodium) content.

Why Gluten Free?

Gluten is a mixture of two proteins that are present in wheat, barley and rye. Gluten causes harmful reactions to people who have celiac disease or are gluten sensitive. But gluten is difficult to avoid, because wheat is the third largest crop in the U.S. (behind corn and soybeans). When wheat, barley and rye acres are combined, more farm acres are used to grow gluten grain crops than any other, with about 4 billion bushels of gluten grains grown in 2011. Because wheat, barley and rye grains are everywhere in our food chain, eating gluten-free involves more complicated than just substituting gluten-free bread for the usual gluten-containing bread for sale on supermarket shelves.

Another problem is gluten cross contamination which occurs when a gluten-free food comes in contact with a food that contains gluten. Cross contamination can happen at a farm where the food is grown, at a manufacturing facility where the food is processed, at a supermarket where a food may be re-packaged, and in your kitchen.

Gluten-free means that a food does not contain the gluten in wheat, barley or rye and sometimes cross-contaminated oats or soy.

The primary reason for a gluten-free diet is to combat celiac disease which is a chronic, systemic, autoimmune disorder that causes intestinal damage. For more on celiac disease see **Appendix A** (page 77).

Another reason to go gluten free is to combat a condition called non-celiac gluten sensitivity that can also affect nearly every system in your body with symptoms that include digestive complaints, skin problems, brain fog, joint pain and numbness in extremities. Still another reason for a gluten-free diet is to combat a wheat allergy. For more on non-celiac gluten sensitivity see Appendix A.

A new reason to go gluten free is that many adults claim that going gluten free not only helped them lose weight but they also felt a lot better. For more on this again see Appendix A.

Is This Diet For You?

The *30-Day Gluten-Free No-Cooking Diet* is for adults:
   - **With celiac disease who want to lose weight.**
   - **With gluten sensitivity or a wheat allergy who want to lose weight.**
   - **Who just want to lose weight and feel better on a gluten-free diet.**
The low-calorie menus assure that you will lose weight, while going gluten free is a healthy bonus that also makes many people feel better while on the diet.

Choose Your Calorie Level

This eBook contains two 30-day diets: a 1200-Calorie diet and a 1500-Calorie diet. And both diets have a meal plan (menu) for each and every one of the 30 days. Which diet calorie level should you choose?

1200-Calorie Diet is appropriate for most women. But due to the relatively low calorie level, you will just barely get all the nutrients and micro nutrients you need – and you also might occasionally feel hungry. (The 1500-Calorie diet might be a better choice for some larger, younger, or more active women.)

1500-Calorie Diet is suitable for most men. This is a reasonable diet calorie level where most adults easily get all the nutrients and micro nutrients they need – and rarely feel hungry. (The 1200-Calorie diet might be a better choice for some smaller, or older, or inactive men.)

Expected Weight Loss

Weight loss occurs when your food energy intake is less than the total energy you expend. This difference in calories is referred to as your calorie deficit. How much weight you lose depends on the magnitude of your calorie deficit. Physiologists have long known that to lose one pound requires a deficit of approximately 3,500 Calories. Therefore, if a person's total calorie deficit over time is known, their weight loss over time can be calculated.

On the *30-Day Gluten-Free No-Cooking Diet*, **most women lose 10 to 15 pounds.** Smaller women, older women and less active women lose a bit less and larger women, younger women and more active women often lose more.

On the *30-Day Gluten-Free No-Cooking Diet*, **most men lose 15 to 20 pounds.** Smaller men, older men and less active men will lose a tad less and larger men, younger men and more active men much more.

Exactly how much weight you will lose depends on how much you weigh, your age and your activity level. For the full story see *Weight Control - U.S. Edition* by Vincent W. Antonetti, Ph.D.

How to Use This eBook

1) Read material in **Appendix A** (page 77): "Gluten Notes" and **Appendix B** (page 80): "Gluten-Free Foods."
2) Choose the calorie level that's right for you, either 1200 or 1500 Calories per day - depending on gender, your size, your age and how active you are.
3) Then to start the diet go to either:
    Day 1 of the 1200-Calorie Diet (page 16)
    Day 1 of the 1500-Calorie Diet.(page 47)

Eat Smart – Gluten Free

First, please read Appendix B "Gluten-Free Foods" which is a listing of many of the gluten-free foods that are available in supermarkets and online.

Then understand that no single food can supply all the nutrients you need in the amounts you need. Gluten free aside for the moment, the most important factors in nutrition are variety, variety, variety! **Variety is the key to a nutritious diet.** As a means of setting strategies for food selection, the U.S. Department of Health and Human Services and the Department of Agriculture issue Dietary Guidelines every five years. The latest Dietary Guidelines describe a healthy diet as one that:

- Emphasizes fruits, vegetables, whole grains, and fat-free or low-fat milk products.
- Includes fish, poultry, lean meats, beans and nuts.
- Is low in saturated fats, trans fats, cholesterol, salt (sodium) and added sugars.

The latest guidelines encourage adults to consume a variety of nutrient-dense foods and beverages within their caloric needs. The afore mentioned U.S. government agencies recommend how much should be eaten from each of the basic food groups. For detailed information on gluten-free eating see Appendix B (page 80).

Even though most adults can get all the vitamins and minerals they need by merely consuming a variety of nutritious foods (from the fruit group, the vegetable group, the grains group, the meat and beans group, the milk group, and the oils group), many physicians recommend a daily multi-vitamin/mineral supplement – just in case you don't eat the way you should.

Be aware that some micronutrients, such as the fat-soluble vitamin A, can be harmful if taken in large quantities. To be safe your multi-vitamin/mineral supplement should contain no more than 100 percent of the recommended dietary allowance (RDA) for each vitamin or mineral. Generally, you don't need the high doses in multi-vitamin/mineral supplements labeled "therapeutic" or "extra-strength." There may be medical reasons for taking larger amounts of a vitamin or mineral than the RDA provides, but check with your doctor first.

Big-Bowl Salad Every Day

Yet another problem with nearly all frozen entrees is that they don't contain enough veggies. The solution is to have a "Big-Bowl Salad" at dinnertime with your frozen entrée. A typical "Big-Bowl Salad" is shown on the following page.

To prepare a "Big-Bowl Salad" start with a relatively large soup bowl (with a volume of at least 24 ounces, or 3 cups). Add about 1½ cups of either green leaf lettuce, Romaine lettuce or a mesclun mix. Then add, as desired, veggies such as broccoli, celery, cucumber, onion, peppers, radish, spinach, tomato, or watercress, to make up the remaining 1½ cups, for a total of 3 cups. This vegetable combination will, on average, total about 100 Calories. You will be eating a "Big-Bowl Salad" every day at dinnertime. Remember that variety is the key to a nutritious diet. So be sure to vary the ingredients of the salad.

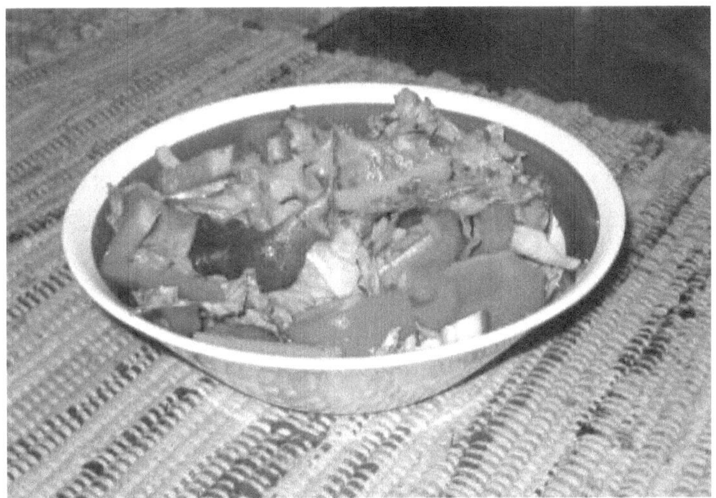

Big-Bowl Salad

Top your "Big-Bowl" with <u>2 tablespoons of any light salad dressing</u> available at your local supermarket that contains no more than 25 Calories per tablespoon. Some of our favorite light salad dressings are:
- **Annie's Lite Raspberry Vinaigrette**
- **Ken's Lite Options Italian w/ Romano & Red Pepper**
- **Newman's Own Lite Red Wine Vinaigrette & Olive Oil**
- **San-J's Tamari Sesame Salad Dressing**

For more gluten-free salad dressing options see page 86. Your "Big-Bowl Salad" with two tablespoons of light salad dressing will cost you roughly 150 Calories but will be packed with lots of health-giving vitamins, minerals and fiber.

About Bread

First appreciate that bread, more specifically whole-grain breads, are good sources of complex carbohydrates and dietary fiber, as well as the B vitamins (thiamin, riboflavin, niacin, and folate), vitamin E, and minerals (iron, magnesium and selenium).

The gluten in wheat, barley and rye consists of two proteins that combine during baking to develop a substance that provides bread with

elasticity and structure. Gluten also helps bread dough rise into a light loaf.
Other grains do not have these characteristics, which is why it is difficult to
find passable gluten-free bread.

The *30-Day Gluten-Free No-Cooking Diet* requires bread at about 70
Calories per slice. These days many supermarkets stock gluten-free bread.
The difficult part is finding a good tasting gluten-free bread with about 70
Calories per slice. The gluten-free breads at your local supermarket vary in
taste and texture, so try different brands of **GF bread** (page 80) before
deciding. As of this writing, our favorite gluten-free bread is Udi's,
particularly Udi's Whole-Grain Bread at about 65 Calories per slice.

Substituting Foods

If there is a food listed in the *30-Day Gluten-Free No-Cooking Diet* that you
don't like, or perhaps that you forgot to pick up while shopping, you probably
can exchange or substitute another food in its place – a technique used by
dieticians. Exchanging a food listed in a diet for another food with
approximately equal caloric value and nutritional content is the foundation of
many successful long-term diets. Substitution possibilities are almost endless
but have to be done carefully. The easiest substitutions are those within the
same food group, such as exchanging one vegetable variety for another, or a
glass of milk for a cup of yogurt. More sophisticated exchanges cross food
groups, such as replacing 3½ ounces of turkey with a tablespoon of peanut
butter on a piece of whole-wheat bread. Both foods are complete protein and
both contain about 175 Calories. With some understanding and experience,
you can substitute foods called for in the *30-Day Gluten-Free No-Cooking
Diet* with equal calorie foods from the same food group.

Breakfast: You may substitute any cereal for any other gluten-free
cereal. For example, if you're not crazy about having Kellogg's Rice
Krispies - gluten-free for breakfast, substitute General Mills Corn Chex, etc.
But remember to adjust the amount of cereal to account for the calorie
difference between brands. (See page 81 for a list of gluten-free cereals.)
And if you don't like the soft-boiled egg called for, cook a fried egg instead.
And if Cantaloupe is on the menu but is not in season, replace cantaloupe
with a half cup of orange juice – both contain about 50 Calories.

Snacks: Again, where 6 ounces of yogurt is specified you may
substitute a 6-ounce glass of skim milk, but to maintain a nutritionally
balanced diet keep this snack a dairy selection. Similarly, when fruit is on
the menu, you may select any type of fruit but do not stray from the fruit
group. Nuts and popcorn can be interchanged at will. Specified convenient
brand-name snacks, such as Skinny Cow ice cream bars and Orville
Redenbacher's Smart Pop Popcorn should be widely available but other

equivalent brands may be substituted if need be. Just make sure the substitute snack has the same calorie count, or very close to the same calorie count, as the specified snack.

Eat Out Once a Week

Everyone deserves a break from the grind of preparing dinner after coming home from work. So one night a week you are encouraged to eat out. There are, however, some rules and caveats involved – these are covered in the next section.

If you would rather not eat out, feel free to have a frozen entree and Big-Bowl salad instead. Just make sure the calorie total for your entree and salad is close to or equal to the calories specified in the daily meal plan for eating out.

Eating Out Challenges

You may eat out once a week. When you're on a gluten-free reducing diet, however, eating in a restaurant can be a double challenge. First, most restaurant portions are huge, easily totaling more than 1000 Calories, and then many restaurants do not offer gluten-free menu selections. On the *30-Day Gluten-Free No-Cooking Diet*, a dinner type (i.e., fish, chicken, etc) and a calorie target are specified. For example Day 7 of the 1200 Calorie diet calls for a chicken dinner and allows you 550 Calories. Follow these tips to make sure your meal is both low calorie, gluten-free and pleasant.

Make sure you choose a restaurant where gluten-free food is available and where you have a fighting chance to achieve your calorie goal. Before you go read the menu online and reduce your food choices so you can have more focused questions for the staff. You are more likely to get a safe meal if you call the restaurant before you go to let them know of your gluten-free needs. And call during a slow time so you can have the host's complete attention.

In the restaurant, to ensure you are served a gluten-free meal, it is important to communicate your need to eat 100 percent gluten-free assertively but amiably. Try to speak directly to the chef or manager. Otherwise, ask your server what is in the food and how it's prepared. Menu descriptions don't always list every ingredient. Try to get a list of ingredients for sauces and dressings. Inquire how gluten-free grains such as rice and risottos are cooked. Sometimes they are cooked in broth which may contain gluten. Confirm that separate, clean utensils and equipment will be used to prepare your meal.

Order something simple, such as broiled fish with steamed vegetables and brown rice. Tell the waiter you want no sauce, no gravy, nothing added.

Then, knowing your calorie objective, and that most fish and chicken are about 50 Calories per ounce, most steamed vegetable servings average approximately 50 Calories per cup, and rice is about 100 Calories per ½ cup, decide how much to eat – and take the remainder home. And consider bringing your own gluten-free salad dressing to the restaurant. If fresh fruit is not an option, pass on dessert and have the evening snack specified in the *30-Day Gluten-Free No-Cooking Diet* meal plan for that day.

Eating Chinese can be especially difficult. Try bringing a restaurant card to the Chinese restaurant. The cards are available online and are designed to help explain a gluten-free diet to a waiter who might not speak English. Rice noodles prepared with vegetables or chicken are generally a safe choice. If you have celiac disease or non-celiac gluten sensitivity, avoid brown sauce which may have a cross-contaminated soy sauce base. Instead, ask for the dish to be prepared with a white sauce using corn starch. And although it is customary to share dishes at a Chinese restaurant, do not permit your dinner companions to contaminate your food. Make sure your friends do not use their gluten-contaminated spoons to serve food from your gluten-free dish.

Social Gatherings can be tricky. At a dinner party, intermingling utensils and serving dishes create a perfect environment for gluten cross contamination, that is for gluten to get in your food. But this does not necessarily mean you should to skip the party. Try to let your host know ahead of time about your gluten-free needs. Do this before your host starts planning the menu. Even better, offer to bring a few dishes to share. This ensures that there will be at least a couple of items you can eat safely and takes a burden off of your host. Finally, ask the host if you can serve yourself first, before serving plates become gluten contaminated.

Important Notes

1) Coffee or tea may be decaf or regular brew. If desired, skim milk and a sugar substitute may be added to coffee or tea. And soy or almond milk may be used instead of cow's milk.

2) Fried eggs and scrambled eggs should be cooked in a pan coated with a non-stick cooking spray. DO NOT USE butter or oil.

3) On bread, corn-on-the-cob, or a baked potato, if desired, you may use a zero-calorie butter substitute spray. (I Can't Believe It's Not Butter spray is gluten free.) DO NOT USE butter or sour cream.

4) Cereals should be selected from the following gluten-free varieties: General Mills Rice Chex, General Mills Corn Chex, General Mills Vanilla Chex, General Mills Cinnamon Chex, General Mills Chocolate Chex, General Mills Apple Cinnamon Chex, General Mills Honey Nut Chex,

Glutino Honey Nut, Glutino Apple Cinnamon, Kellogg's Rice Krispies - gluten-free, Bob's Red Mill Oat Meal and Gifts of Nature (Montana) Oat Meal. Always use skim milk in your cereal.

5) <u>Bread:</u> Udi's Whole Grain Bread is a good choice and has 65 Calories per slice. These days many supermarkets stock gluten-free bread although you often can find a better selection online. If desired, bread may be sprayed with a zero-calorie butter substitute. DO NOT USE butter.

6) Use only lean cuts of meat trimmed of all visible fat. Poultry should be limited to chicken or turkey breasts (white meat and skinless only).

7) When canned tuna or salmon is specified, use only fish packed in water.

8) When a GF cookie is specified, choose from a selection ranging from 40 to 90 Calories per cookie.

9) An unlimited amount of green salad may be eaten, but the GF salad dressing should be as specified On page 86. (Note, in the meal plans Evoo means extra virgin olive oil.)

10) Use freely as desired: clear unsweetened coffee, clear unsweetened tea, water, seltzer water, any diet soda, clear soups without fat, bouillon, and seasonings such as mustard, cinnamon, dill, herbs, red and black pepper, curry and vinegar.

11) On days when a leftover is specified for lunch. Eat about half as much as you ate for dinner a night or two before.

12) Any specified snack may be moved to any other part of the day, and/or combined with lunch or dinner.

13) Although it's recommended that you follow the diet days as specified, it's fine to occasionally skip a day and/or pick and choose the days you prefer. (Nutritionally, each day stands on its own.)

14) After you complete the 30th day on the diet, if you want to lose more weight you may repeat the diet by starting over at Day 1.

Keeping It Off

Within five years, more than 90 percent of all dieters regain every pound they have lost. Why? In most cases it's because after losing weight most people eventually revert to their pre-diet eating and exercising habits, and this inevitably leads to their regaining the weight they lost – and often more. Obviously after a diet you weigh less. The fact is the less you weigh, the less you need to eat to sustain your lower weight.

A study, published in the *Annals of Internal Medicine*, that followed 4,000 people for three decades suggests that in the long term, 90 percent of men and 70 percent of women will become overweight. Interestingly, half of the men and women in the study, who had made it well into adulthood without a weight problem, ultimately also became overweight and a third actually became obese. The point being that you can never become complacent. You must continually watch your weight because we are all at risk of becoming overweight.

The key to long-term weight control success is knowledge and understanding, combined of course with desire and self-discipline. Once you reach your weight goal, we suggest you read ***Weight Maintenance - U.S. Edition*** by Vincent Antonetti, Ph.D. (also published by NoPaperPress) – absolutely the best weight maintenance book, or eBook, on the market.

1200 Calorie Daily Menus

Day 1 – 1200 Calorie Diet

BREAKFAST	Calories	Totals
Orange juice (½ cup)	50	
Fried egg	80	
GF raisin bread toasted (1 slice) (page 80)	70	
Coffee (Notes page 12)	10	210 Cal
.		
SNACK		
Coffee or tea	10	10 Cal
LUNCH		
Soup (See Appendix D - page 89)	150	
GF bread (1 slice)	70	
Lettuce & tomato w 1 Tbsp lite GF dressing*	45	
Canned pineapple (½ cup, no-sugar-added	40	
Water	0	305 Cal
*See page 86.		
SNACK		
GF yogurt (6 oz, nonfat, any flavor) (page 85)	90	
Coffee or tea	10	100 Cal
DINNER		
Frozen dinner (See Appendix C - page 88)*	300	
"Big-Bowl Salad" (See page 8 for ingredients)	150	
Water with lemon wedge	10	460 Cal
* See page 85 for additional frozen-entree choices.		
SNACK		
Skinny Cow Low Fat Bar (any flavor)*	100	
Coffee or tea	10	110 Cal
* Ice cream		1195 Cal

Day 2 – 1200 Calorie Diet

BREAKFAST	Calories	Totals
Fresh or frozen strawberries (½ cup)	25	
Van's Waffles (2) original or blueberry (page 81)	210	
Light GF Pancake Syrup (1½ Tbsp) (page 87)	40	
Coffee (Notes page 12)	10	285 Cal
SNACK		
Coffee or tea	10	10 Cal
LUNCH		
Ham* (2 oz) w mustard on 2 slices GF bread	300	
Fresh fruit in season (apple, peach, etc)	70	
Coffee or tea	10	380 Cal
* See page 84.		
SNACK		
GF yogurt* (6 oz, nonfat, any flavor)	90	
Coffee or tea	10	100 Cal
* See page 85.		
DINNER		
Frozen dinner (Appendix C - page 88)	260	
"Big-Bowl Salad" (See page 8 for ingredients)	150	
Water with lemon wedge	10	420 Cal
SNACK		
Coffee or tea	10	10 Cal
		1205 Cal

Day 3 – 1200 Calorie Diet

BREAKFAST	Calories	Totals
Grapefruit (½)	75	
Scrambled egg	80	
Gluten-free (GF) bread toasted (1 slice)	70	
Coffee	10	235 Cal
SNACK		
Coffee or tea	10	10 Cal
LUNCH		
Soup (Appendix D - page 89)	140	
GF yogurt (6 oz, nonfat, any flavor) (page 85)	90	
Coffee or tea	10	240 Cal
SNACK		
Fresh fruit in season (apple, plum, etc)	70	
Coffee or tea	10	80 Cal
DINNER		
Frozen dinner (Appendix C - page 88)	200	
"Big-Bowl Salad"	150	
GF bread (1 slice)	70	
Water with lemon wedge	10	430 Cal
SNACK		
Raw Revolution Peanut Butter Chocolate Bar*	200	
Coffee or tea	10	210 Cal
* See page 83.		1205 Cal

Day 4 – 1200 Calorie Diet

BREAKFAST	Calories	Totals
Grapefruit (½)	75	
Rice Chex* (1 cup) + ½ cup milk* + ½ banana	195	
Coffee	10	280 Cal
* Always use skim milk. See Note 1 on page 12.		
SNACK		
Coffee or tea	10	10 Cal
LUNCH		
GF Cottage cheese* (1 cup no fat)	140	
Fresh fruit in season (peach, plum, etc)	70	
GF bread (1 slice)	70	
Hot or iced tea	10	290 Cal
* Cabot No-Fat Cottage Cheese is gluten free		
SNACK		
Coffee or tea	10	10 Cal
DINNER		
Frozen dinner (Appendix C - page 88)	270	
"Big-Bowl Salad"	150	
GF bread (1 slice)	70	
Water with lemon wedge	10	500 Cal
SNACK		
Handful unsalted mixed nuts*	100	
Coffee or tea	10	110 Cal
* See page 85.		1200 Cal

Day 5 – 1200 Calorie Diet

BREAKFAST	Calories	Totals
Cantaloupe (½ medium)	50	
Fried egg	80	
GF raisin bread - toasted (1 slice)	70	
Coffee	10	210 Cal
SNACK		
Fresh fruit in season (peach, plum, etc)	70	
Coffee or tea	10	80 Cal
LUNCH		
Soup (Appendix D - page 89)*	260	
GF bread (1 slice)	70	
Water	0	330 Cal
* Enjoy 2 servings of a 130 Cal soup.		
SNACK		
GF yogurt (6 oz, nonfat, any flavor) (page 85)	90	
Coffee or tea	10	100 Cal
DINNER		
Frozen dinner (Appendix C - page 88)	330	
"Big-Bowl Salad"	150	
Water	0	480 Cal
SNACK		
Coffee or tea	10	10 Cal
		1210

Day 6 – 1200 Calorie Diet

BREAKFAST	Calories	Totals
Orange juice (½ cup)	50	
Rice Krispies* (1 cup) + ½ cup milk + 1 Tbsp raisins	200	
Coffee	10	260 Cal
* Gluten-free variety. Always use skim milk!		
SNACK		
Coffee or tea	10	10 Cal
LUNCH		
Salad (3 oz canned tuna* 1 tsp Evoo onions, celery)	175	
Lettuce & tomato wedges	20	
GF bread (1 slice)	70	
Fresh fruit in season (apple, peach, etc)	70	
Diet soda (or water)	0	335 Cal
* See page 84.		
SNACK		
Coffee or tea	10	10 Cal
DINNER		
Frozen dinner (Appendix C - page 88)	240	
"Big-Bowl Salad"	150	
GF bread (1 slice)	70	
Hot or ice tea	10	470 Cal
SNACK		
GF Popcorn - Mini Bag (page 85)	100	
Coffee or tea	10	110 Cal
		1195 Cal

Day 7 – 1200 Calorie Diet

BREAKFAST	Calories	Totals
Cantaloupe (½ medium)	50	
GF Oatmeal* (½ cup dry) + ½ cup skim milk	190	
Coffee	10	250 Cal
* See page 81.		
SNACK		
Coffee or tea	10	10 Cal
LUNCH		
Udi's Margherita Pizza (half of GF 9-inch pizza)*	300	
Diet soda or water	0	300 Cal
* Freeze the remaining half for Day 14 lunch.		
SNACK		
Fresh fruit in season (apple, peach, etc)	70	
Coffee or tea	10	80 Cal
DINNER		
Eat Out – Chicken dinner (See page 11)		
Max allowable calories	550	550 Cal
SNACK		
Coffee or tea	10	10 Cal
		1200 Cal

Day 8 – 1200 Calorie Diet

BREAKFAST	Calories	Totals
Orange juice (½ cup)	50	
Cinnamon Chex (¾ cup) + ½ cup milk + ½ banana	215	
Coffee	10	275 Cal
SNACK		
Coffee or tea	10	10 Cal
LUNCH		
Soup (Appendix D - page 89)	110	
GF bread (1 slice)	70	
Fresh fruit in season (apple, plum, etc)	70	
Coffee or tea	10	260 Cal
SNACK		
Coffee or tea	10	10 Cal
DINNER		
Frozen dinner (Appendix C - page 88)	290	
"Big-Bowl Salad"	150	
GF cookie*	90	
Coffee or tea	10	540 Cal
* See page 83.		
SNACK		
GF Popcorn - Mini Bag (page 85)	100	
Coffee or tea	10	110 Cal
		1205 Cal

Day 9 – 1200 Calorie Diet

BREAKFAST	Calories	Totals
Fresh or frozen strawberries (½ cup)	25	
Van's Waffles (2) - original or blueberry	210	
Light GF Pancake Syrup* (1½ Tbsp) (page 87)	40	
Coffee	10	285 Cal
SNACK		
Coffee or tea	10	10 Cal
LUNCH		
Ham* (2 oz) with mustard on 2 slices GF bread	290	
Fresh fruit in season (pear, plum, etc)	70	
Coffee or tea	10	370 Cal
* See page 84.		
SNACK		
GF yogurt (6 oz, nonfat, any flavor)	90	
Coffee or tea	10	100 Cal
DINNER		
Frozen dinner (Appendix C - page 88)	250	
"Big-Bowl Salad"	150	
Water with lemon wedge	10	410 Cal
SNACK		
Coffee or tea	10	10 Cal
		1185 Cal

Day 10 – 1200 Calorie Diet

BREAKFAST	Calories	Totals
Grapefruit (½)	75	
Soft-boiled egg (1)	80	
GF bread - toasted (1 slice)	70	
Coffee	10	235 Cal
SNACK		
Coffee or tea	10	10 Cal
LUNCH		
Soup (Appendix D - page 89)	180	
GF bread (1 slice)	70	
Coffee or tea	10	260 Cal
SNACK		
Coffee or tea	10	10 Cal
DINNER		
Frozen dinner (Appendix C - page 88)	350	
"Big-Bowl Salad"	150	
Fresh fruit in season (apple, plum, etc)	70	
Water with lemon wedge	10	580 Cal
SNACK		
Skinny Cow Low Fat Ice Cream Bar (any flavor)	100	
Coffee or tea	10	110 Cal
		1205 Cal

Day 11 – 1200 Calorie Diet

BREAKFAST	Calories	Totals
Grapefruit (½)	**75**	
Rice Chex (1 cup) + ½ cup skim milk + ½ banana	**195**	
Coffee	**10**	**280 Cal**
SNACK		
Coffee or tea	**10**	**10 Cal**
LUNCH		
GF Cottage cheese* (1 cup no fat)	**140**	
Fresh fruit in season (apple, peach, etc)	**70**	
GF bread (1 slice)	**70**	
Hot or iced tea	**10**	**290 Cal**
* Cabot No-Fat Cottage Cheese is gluten free		
SNACK		
GF Ginger-Snap cookie (See page 83)	**40**	
Coffee or tea	**10**	**50 Cal**
DINNER		
Frozen dinner (Appendix C - page 88)	**240**	
"Big-Bowl Salad"	**150**	
Whole-grain bread (1 slice)	**70**	
Water with lemon wedge	**10**	**470 Cal**
SNACK		
Handful unsalted mixed nuts (page 85)	**100**	
Coffee or tea	**10**	**110 Cal**
		1210 Cal

Day 12 – 1200 Calorie

BREAKFAST	Calories	Totals
Orange juice (½ cup)	50	
Scrambled egg	80	
GF bread - toasted (1 slice)	70	
Coffee	10	210 Cal
SNACK		
GF yogurt (6 oz, nonfat, any flavor)	90	
Coffee or tea	10	100 Cal
LUNCH		
Soup (Appendix D - page 89)	160	
Coffee or tea	10	170 Cal
SNACK		
Fresh fruit in season (apple, plum, etc)	70	
Coffee or tea	10	80 Cal
DINNER		
Frozen dinner (Appendix C - page 88)	370	
"Big-Bowl Salad"	150	
GF bread (1 slice)	70	
Water with lemon wedge	10	600 Cal
SNACK		
GF Ginger-Snap cookie (page 83)	40	
Coffee or tea	10	50 Cal
		1205 Cal

Day 13 – 1200 Calorie

BREAKFAST	Calories	Totals
Orange juice (½ cup)	50	
Rice Krispies* (1 cup) + ½ cup milk + 1 Tbsp raisins	200	
Coffee	10	260 Cal
* Gluten-free variety		
SNACK		
Coffee or tea	10	10 Cal
LUNCH		
Peanut butter* (2 Tbsp) on 2 slices GF bread	330	
Skim milk (4 oz)	45	
Fresh fruit in season (peach, plum, etc)	70	
Water	0	445 Cal
* See page 85.		
SNACK		
Coffee or tea	10	10 Cal
DINNER		
Frozen dinner (Appendix C - page 88)	200	
"Big-Bowl Salad"	150	
Diet soda or water	0	350 Cal
SNACK		
GF Cookies (2) (page 83)	120	
Coffee or tea	10	130 Cal
		1205 Cal

Day 14 – 1200 Calorie

BREAKFAST	Calories	Totals
Cantaloupe (½ medium)	50	
Oatmeal (½ cup dry) + ½ cup milk + 1 Tbsp raisins	230	
Coffee	10	290 Cal
SNACK		
Coffee or tea	10	10 Cal
LUNCH		
Udi's Margherita Pizza*	300	
Diet soda (or water)	0	300 Cal
* This is leftover pizza from Day 7.		
SNACK		
Fresh fruit in season (apple, peach, etc)	70	
Coffee or tea	10	80 Cal
DINNER		
Eat Out – Chicken dinner		
Max allowable calories	510	510 Cal
SNACK		
Coffee or tea	10	10 Cal
		1200 Cal

Day 15 – 1200 Calorie

BREAKFAST	Calories	Totals
Fresh sliced orange	75	
Cinnamon Chex (¾ cup) + ½ cup milk + ½ banana	215	
Coffee	10	300 Cal
SNACK		
Handful unsalted mixed nuts	100	
Coffee or tea	10	110 Cal
LUNCH		
Soup (Appendix D - page 89)	90	
GF bread (1 slice)	70	
Coffee or tea	10	170 Cal
SNACK		
Fresh fruit in season (apple, plum, etc)	70	
Coffee or tea	10	80 Cal
DINNER		
Frozen dinner (Appendix C - page 88)	320	
"Big-Bowl Salad".(See page 8 for ingredients)	150	
Water with lemon wedge	10	480 Cal
SNACK		
GF Cookie	60	
Coffee or tea	10	70 Cal
		1210 Cal

Day 16 – 1200 Calorie

BREAKFAST	Calories	Totals
Cantaloupe (½ medium)	50	
Rice Chex (1 cup) + ½ cup milk* + ½ banana	195	
Coffee	10	255 Cal
* Always use skim milk in cereal!		
SNACK		
Coffee or tea	10	10 Cal
LUNCH		
Soup (Appendix D - page 89)	100	
GF bread (1 slice)	70	
Fresh fruit in season (apple, plum, etc)	70	
Water	0	240 Cal
SNACK		
Handful unsalted mixed nuts	100	
Coffee or tea	10	110 Cal
DINNER		
Frozen dinner (Appendix C - page 88)	240	
"Big-Bowl Salad"	150	
Water	0	390 Cal
SNACK		
Raw Revolution Peanut Butter Chocolate Bar	200	
Coffee or tea	10	210 Cal
		1205 Cal

Day 17 – 1200 Calorie

BREAKFAST	Calories	Totals
Orange juice (½ cup)	50	
Fried egg	80	
GF bread - toasted (1 slice)	70	
Coffee	10	210 Cal
SNACK		
GF yogurt (6 oz, nonfat, any flavor)	90	
Coffee or tea	10	100 Cal
LUNCH		
Soup (Appendix D - page 89)	160	
GF bread (1 slice)	70	
Coffee or tea	10	240 Cal
SNACK		
Fresh fruit in season (pear, plum, etc)	70	
Coffee or tea	10	80 Cal
DINNER		
Frozen dinner (Appendix C - page 88)	280	
"Big-Bowl Salad"	150	
Water with lemon wedge	10	440 Cal
SNACK		
GF Popcorn - Mini Bag	100	
Coffee or tea	10	110 Cal
		1180 Cal

Day 18 – 1200 Calorie

BREAKFAST	Calories	Totals
Grapefruit (½)	75	
Rice Krispies* (1 cup) + ½ cup milk + 1 Tbsp raisins	200	
Coffee	10	285 Cal
* Gluten-free variety		
SNACK		
Coffee or tea	10	10 Cal
LUNCH		
Cottage cheese (1 cup no fat)	140	
Fresh fruit in season (apple, plum, etc)	70	
GF Bread (1 slice)	70	
Water	0	280 Cal
SNACK		
GF Popcorn - Mini Bag (page 85)	100	
Coffee or tea	10	110 Cal
DINNER		
Frozen dinner (Appendix C - page 88)	310	
"Big-Bowl Salad"	150	
GF bread (1 slice)	70	
Water	0	530 Cal
SNACK		
Coffee or tea	10	10 Cal
		1225 Cal

Day 19 – 1200 Calorie

BREAKFAST	Calories	Totals
Grapefruit (½)	75	
Fried egg	80	
GF bread - toasted (1 slice)	70	
Coffee	10	235 Cal
SNACK		
GF yogurt (6 oz, nonfat, any flavor)	90	
Coffee or tea	10	100 Cal
LUNCH		
Soup (Appendix D - page 89)	200	
GF bread (1 slice)	70	
Coffee or tea	10	280 Cal
SNACK		
Coffee or tea	10	10 Cal
DINNER		
Frozen dinner (Appendix C - page 88)	350	
"Big-Bowl Salad"	150	
Fresh fruit in season (apple, pear, etc)	70	
Diet soda	0	570 Cal
SNACK		
Coffee or tea	10	10 Cal
		1205 Cal

Day 20 - 1200 Calorie

BREAKFAST	Calories	Totals
Fresh or frozen strawberries (½ cup)	25	
Van's Waffles (2) - original or blueberry	210	
Light GF Pancake Syrup (1½ Tbsp) (page 87)	40	
Coffee	10	285 Cal
SNACK		
Coffee or tea	10	10 Cal
LUNCH		
Soup (Appendix D - page 89)	160	
GF bread (1 slice)	70	
Hot or Ice Tea	10	240 Cal
SNACK		
GF yogurt (6 oz, nonfat, any flavor)	90	
Coffee or tea	10	100 Cal
DINNER		
Frozen dinner (Appendix C - page 88)	290	
"Big-Bowl Salad"	150	
GF bread (1 slice)	70	
Water	0	510 Cal
SNACK		
Fresh fruit in season (apple, plum, etc)	70	
Coffee or tea	10	80 Cal
		1225 Cal

<u>Day 21 - 1200 Calorie</u>

<u>BREAKFAST</u>	**<u>Calories</u>**	**<u>Totals</u>**
Cantaloupe (½ medium)	50	
Oatmeal (½ cup dry) + ½ cup skim milk	190	
Coffee	10	250 Cal
<u>SNACK</u>		
Coffee or tea	10	10 Cal
<u>LUNCH</u>		
Salad (3 oz canned tuna, 1 tsp Evoo, onions, celery)	175	
Lettuce & tomato wedges	20	
GF bread (1 slice)	70	
Diet soda (or water)	0	265 Cal
<u>SNACK</u>		
GF Popcorn - Mini Bag	100	
Coffee or tea	10	110 Cal
<u>DINNER</u>		
Eat Out – Chicken dinner		
Max allowable calories	550	550 Cal
<u>SNACK</u>		
Coffee or tea	10	10 Cal
		1195 Cal

Day 22 - 1200 Calorie

BREAKFAST	Calories	Totals
Cantaloupe (½ medium)	50	
Cinnamon Chex (¾ cup) + ½ cup milk + ½ banana	215	
Coffee	10	310 Cal
SNACK		
Coffee or tea	10	10 Cal
LUNCH		
Soup (Appendix D - page 89)	150	
GF bread (1 slice)	70	
Coffee or tea	10	230 Cal
SNACK		
Coffee or tea	10	10 Cal
DINNER		
Frozen dinner (Appendix C - page 88)	330	
"Big-Bowl Salad"	150	
GF bread (1 slice)	70	
Water with lemon wedge	10	560 Cal
SNACK		
Fresh fruit in season (apple, peach, etc)	70	
Coffee or tea	10	80 Cal
		1200 Cal

Day 23 – 1200 Calorie

BREAKFAST	Calories	Totals
Fresh or frozen strawberries (½ cup)	25	
Van's Waffles (2) - original or blueberry	210	
Light GF Pancake Syrup (1½ Tbsp)	40	
Coffee	10	285 Cal
SNACK		
Coffee or tea	10	10 Cal
LUNCH		
Ham (2 oz) with mustard on 2 slices GF bread	300	
Fresh fruit in season (pear, peach, etc)	70	
Coffee or tea	10	380 Cal
SNACK		
GF yogurt (6 oz, nonfat, any flavor)	90	
Coffee or tea	10	100 Cal
DINNER		
Frozen dinner (Appendix C - page 88)	250	
"Big-Bowl Salad"	150	
Water with lemon wedge	10	410 Cal
SNACK		
Coffee or tea	10	10 Cal
		1195 Cal

Day 24 – 1200 Calorie

BREAKFAST	Calories	Totals
Orange juice (½ cup)	50	
Soft-boiled egg	80	
GF bread - toasted (1 slice)	70	
Coffee	10	210 Cal
SNACK		
GF yogurt (6 oz any flavor)	90	
Coffee or tea	10	100 Cal
LUNCH		
Soup (Appendix D - page 89)	180	
GF bread (1 slice)	70	
Coffee or tea	10	260 Cal
SNACK		
Fresh fruit in season (apple, plum, etc)	70	
Coffee or tea	10	80 Cal
DINNER		
Frozen dinner (Appendix C - page 88)	290	
"Big-Bowl Salad"	150	
Water with lemon wedge	10	450 Cal
SNACK		
GF Cookie (page 83)	90	
Coffee or tea	10	100 Cal
		1200 Cal

Day 25 – 1200 Calorie

BREAKFAST	Calories	Totals
Fresh sliced orange	75	
Rice Chex (1 cup) + ½ cup milk* + ½ banana	195	
Coffee	10	280 Cal
* Always use skim milk!		
SNACK		
Coffee or tea	10	10 Cal
LUNCH		
Cottage cheese (1 cup no fat)	140	
Fresh fruit in season (apple, plum, etc)	70	
GF Bread (1 slice)	70	
Hot or ice tea	10	290 Cal
SNACK		
Coffee or tea	10	10 Cal
DINNER		
Frozen dinner (Appendix C - page 88)	280	
"Big-Bowl Salad"	150	
GF Bread (1 slice)	70	
Water	0	500 Cal
SNACK		
Handful unsalted mixed nuts	100	
Coffee or tea	10	110 Cal
		1200 Cal

Day 26 – 1200 Calorie

BREAKFAST	Calories	Totals
Cantaloupe (½ medium)	50	
Fried egg	80	
Toasted GF bread (1 slice)	70	
Coffee	10	210 Cal
SNACK		
GF yogurt (6 oz, nonfat, any flavor)	90	
Coffee or tea	10	100 Cal
LUNCH		
Soup (Appendix D - page 89)	200	
GF bread (1 slice)	70	
Fresh fruit in season (apple, plum, etc)	70	
Water with lemon wedge	10	350 Cal
SNACK		
Coffee or tea	10	10 Cal
DINNER		
Frozen dinner (Appendix C - page 88)	240	
"Big-Bowl Salad"	150	
Water with lemon wedge	10	400 Cal
SNACK		
Skinny Cow Low Fat Bar (any flavor)	100	
Coffee or tea	10	110 Cal
		1180 Cal

Day 27 – 1200 Calorie

BREAKFAST	Calories	Totals
Cantaloupe (½ medium)	50	
Oatmeal (½ cup dry) + ½ cup milk + 1 Tbsp raisins	220	
Coffee	10	280 Cal
SNACK		
Fresh fruit in season (peach, plum, etc)	70	70 Cal
LUNCH		
Peanut butter (2 Tbsp) on 2 slices GF bread	330	
Skim milk (4 oz)	45	
Water	0	375 Cal
SNACK		
Coffee or tea	10	10 Cal
DINNER		
Frozen dinner (Appendix C - page 88)	310	
"Big-Bowl Salad"	150	
Water	0	460 Cal
SNACK		
Coffee or tea	10	10 Cal
		1205 Cal

Day 28 – 1200 Calorie

BREAKFAST	Calories	Totals
Orange juice (½ cup)	50	
Rice Krispies* (1 cup) + ½ cup milk + 1 Tbsp raisins	200	
Coffee	10	260 Cal
* Gluten-free variety		
SNACK		
Coffee or tea	10	10 Cal
LUNCH		
Salad (3 oz canned tuna,1 tsp Evoo, onions, celery)	175	
Lettuce & tomato wedges	20	
GF bread (1 slice)	70	
Diet soda (or water)	0	265 Cal
SNACK		
Fresh fruit in season (pear, plum, etc)	70	
Coffee or tea	10	80
DINNER		
Eat Out – Fish dinner		
Max allowable calories	575	575 Cal
SNACK		
Coffee or tea	10	10 Cal
		1200

Day 29 – 1200 Calorie

BREAKFAST	Calories	Totals
Orange juice (½ cup)	50	
Rice Chex (1 cup) + ½ cup milk + ½ banana	195	
Coffee	10	255 Cal
SNACK		
Coffee or tea	10	10 Cal
LUNCH		
Soup (Appendix D - page 89)	140	
GF bread (1 slice)	70	
Coffee or tea	10	220 Cal
SNACK		
GF Popcorn - Mini Bag	100	
Coffee or tea	10	110 Cal
DINNER		
Frozen dinner (Appendix C - page 88)	270	
"Big-Bowl Salad"	150	
Fresh fruit in season (apple, plum, etc)	70	
Water with lemon wedge	10	500 Cal
SNACK		
GF Cookie	90	
Coffee or tea	10	100 Cal
		1195 Cal

<h1 style="text-align:center">Day 30 – 1200 Calorie</h1>

BREAKFAST	Calories	Totals
Fresh or frozen strawberries (½ cup)	25	
Van's Waffles (2) - original or blueberry	210	
Light Pancake Syrup (1½ Tbsp)	40	
Coffee	10	285 Cal
SNACK		
GF yogurt (6 oz, nonfat, any flavor)	90	
Coffee or tea	10	100 Cal
LUNCH		
Ham (2 oz) with mustard on 2 slices GF bread	290	
Fresh fruit in season (peach, plum, etc)	70	
Coffee or tea	10	370 Cal
SNACK		
Coffee or tea	10	10 Cal
DINNER		
Frozen dinner (Appendix C - page 88)	270	
"Big-Bowl Salad"	150	
Water with lemon wedge	10	430 Cal
SNACK		
Coffee or tea	10	10 Cal
		1205 Cal

1500 Calorie Daily Menus

Day 1 – 1500 Calorie Diet

BREAKFAST	Calories	Total
Orange juice (½ cup)	50	
Fried egg	80	
GF Turkey bacon (1 slice) (page 84)	35	
GF raisin bread toasted (1 slice) (page 80)	70	
Coffee (Notes - page 12)	10	245 Cal
SNACK		
GF yogurt (6 oz, nonfat, any flavor) (page 85)	90	
Coffee or tea	10	100 Cal
LUNCH		
Soup (See Appendix D - page 89)	150	
GF bread (1 slice)	70	
Lettuce & tomato w 1 Tbsp lite GF dressing*	45	
Canned pineapple (½ cup, no-sugar-added juice)	40	
Water	0	305 Cal
* See page 86.		
SNACK		
Handful unsalted mixed nuts (page 85)	100	
Coffee or tea	10	110 Cal
DINNER		
Frozen dinner (See Appendix C - page 88)	300	
"Big-Bowl Salad".(See page 8 for ingredients)	150	
Fresh fruit in season (apple, peach, etc)	70	
Water with lemon wedge	10	530 Cal
SNACK		
Raw Revolution Peanut Butter Chocolate Bar*	200	
Coffee or tea	10	210 Cal
* See page 83.		1500 Cal

Day 2 – 1500 Calorie Diet

BREAKFAST	Calories	Totals
Fresh or frozen strawberries (½ cup)	25	
Van's Waffles (2) - original or blueberry	210	
GF Turkey Breakfast Sausage Links* (2)	50	
Light Pancake Syrup** (2 Tbsp)	50	
Coffee	10	345 Cal
* See page 84. **See page 87.		
SNACK		
GF yogurt (6 oz, nonfat, any flavor)	90	
Coffee or tea	10	100 Cal
LUNCH		
Ham* (2 oz) w mustard on 2 slices GF bread	300	
Fresh fruit in season (apple, peach, etc)	70	
Hot or iced tea	10	380 Cal
* See page 84.		
SNACK		
Handful unsalted mixed nuts	100	
Coffee or tea	10	110 Cal
DINNER		
Frozen dinner (Appendix C - page 88)	260	
"Big-Bowl Salad".(See page 8 for ingredients)	150	
Water with lemon wedge	10	420 Cal
SNACK		
GF cookie (2 cookies) (page 83)	130	
Coffee or tea	10	140 Cal
		1505 Cal

Day 3 – 1500 Calorie Diet

BREAKFAST	Calories	Totals
Grapefruit (½)	75	
Scrambled eggs (2)	160	
GF Turkey bacon (3 slices) (page 84)	105	
GF bread toasted (1 slice)	70	
Coffee	10	420 Cal
SNACK		
GF yogurt (6 oz, nonfat, any flavor)	90	
Coffee or tea	10	100 Cal
LUNCH		
Soup (Appendix D - page 89)	140	
Fresh fruit in season (pear, peach, etc)	70	
Coffee or tea	10	240 Cal
* See Appendix D for note regarding serving size		
SNACK		
Handful unsalted mixed nuts	100	
Coffee or tea	10	110 Cal
DINNER		
Frozen dinner (Appendix C - page 88)	200	
"Big-Bowl Salad"	150	
GF bread (1 slice)	70	
Water	0	420 Cal
SNACK		
Raw Revolution Peanut Butter Chocolate Bar*	200	
Coffee or tea	10	210 Cal
* See page 83.		1500 Cal

Day 4 – 1500 Calorie Diet

BREAKFAST	Calories	Totals
Grapefruit (½)	75	
Rice Chex* (1 cup) + ½ cup milk+ ½ banana	245	
Coffee	10	330 Cal
* See page 81 for more GF cereals.		
SNACK		
Handful unsalted mixed nuts	100	
Coffee or tea	10	110 Cal
LUNCH		
GF Cottage cheese* (1 cup no fat) (page 85)	140	
Fresh fruit in season (apple, plum, etc)	70	
GF bread (1 slice)	70	
Hot or iced tea	10	290 Cal
* Cabot No-Fat Cottage Cheese is gluten free		
SNACK		
GF Popcorn - Mini Bag (page 85)	100	
Coffee or tea	10	110 Cal
DINNER		
Frozen dinner (Appendix C - page 88)	270	
"Big-Bowl Salad"	150	
GF bread (1 slice)	70	
Water with lemon wedge	10	500 Cal
SNACK		
GF cookie* (2 cookies)	130	
Coffee or tea	10	140 Cal
* See page 83.		1480 Cal

Day 5 – 1500 Calorie Diet

BREAKFAST	Calories	Totals
Cantaloupe (½ medium)	50	
Fried egg	80	
GF Turkey bacon (3 slices)	105	
GF raisin bread - toasted (2 slices)	140	
Coffee	10	385 Cal
SNACK		
Fresh fruit in season (apple, peach, etc)	70	
Coffee or tea	10	80 Cal
LUNCH		
Soup (Appendix D - page 89)*	260	
GF bread (1 slice)	70	
Hot or ice tea	10	340 Cal
* Enjoy 2 servings of a 130 Cal soup.		
SNACK		
GF yogurt (6 oz, nonfat, any flavor)	90	
Coffee or tea	10	100 Cal
DINNER		
Frozen dinner (Appendix C - page 88)	330	
"Big-Bowl Salad"	150	
Water with lemon wedge	10	490 Cal
SNACK		
Skinny Cow Low Fat Bar (any flavor)*	100	
Coffee or tea	10	110 Cal
* Ice cream		1505 Cal

Day 6 – 1500 Calorie Diet

BREAKFAST	Calories	Totals
Orange juice (½ cup)	50	
Rice Krispies* (1 cup) + ½ cup milk + 1 Tbsp raisins	200	
Coffee	10	260 Cal
* Gluten-free variety		
SNACK		
Handful unsalted mixed nuts	100	
Coffee or tea	10	110 Cal
LUNCH		
Salad (3 oz canned tuna* 1 tsp Evoo onions, celery)	175	
Lettuce & tomato wedges	20	
GF bread (1 slice)	70	
Fresh fruit in season (apple, peach, etc)	70	
Hot or ice tea	10	345 Cal
SNACK		
GF Popcorn - Mini Bag (page 85)	100	
Coffee or tea	10	110 Cal
DINNER		
Frozen dinner (Appendix C - page 88)	240	
"Big-Bowl Salad"	150	
GF bread (1 slice)	70	
GF cookie (page 83)	90	
Hot or ice tea	10	560 Cal
SNACK		
Skinny Cow Low Fat Ice Cream Bar (any flavor)	100	
Coffee or tea	10	110 Cal
		1495 Cal

DAY 7 – 1500 Calorie Diet

BREAKFAST	Calories	Totals
Cantaloupe (½ medium)	50	
GF Oatmeal* (½ cup dry) + ½ cup skim milk	190	
Coffee	10	250 Cal
* See page 81.		
SNACK		
Fresh fruit in season (apple, peach, etc)	70	
Coffee or tea	10	80 Cal
LUNCH		
Udi's Margherita Pizza (half of GF 9-inch pizza)*	300	
Diet soda or water	0	300 Cal
* Freeze the remaining pizza half for Day 14 lunch.		
SNACK		
Handful unsalted mixed nuts	100	
Coffee or tea	10	110 Cal
DINNER		
Eat Out – Chicken dinner*		
Max allowable calories	650	650
* See page 11 for eating out tips.		
SNACK		
GF yogurt (6 oz, nonfat, any flavor)	90	
Coffee or tea	10	100 Cal
		1490 Cal

DAY 8 – 1500 Calorie Diet

BREAKFAST	Calories	Totals
Orange juice (½ cup)	50	
Cinnamon Chex (¾ cup) + ½ cup milk + ½ banana	215	
Coffee	10	275 Cal
* Always use skim milk.		
SNACK		
Handful unsalted mixed nuts	100	
Coffee or tea	10	110 Cal
LUNCH		
Soup (Appendix D - page 89)	110	
GF bread (1 slice)	70	
Fresh fruit in season (peach, plum, etc)	70	
Coffee or tea	10	260 Cal
SNACK		
GF Popcorn - Mini Bag	100	
Coffee or tea	10	110 Cal
DINNER		
Frozen dinner (Appendix C - page 88)	290	
"Big-Bowl Salad"	150	
GF cookie (page 83)	90	
Coffee or tea	10	540 Cal
SNACK		
Raw Revolution Peanut Butter Chocolate Bar	200	
Coffee or tea	10	210 Cal
		1505 Cal

DAY 9 – 1500 Calorie Diet

BREAKFAST	Calories	Totals
Fresh or frozen strawberries (½ cup)	25	
Van's Waffles (2) - original or blueberry	210	
GF Turkey Breakfast Sausage Links (2)	50	
Light Pancake Syrup (2 Tbsp) (page 87)	50	
Coffee	10	345 Cal
SNACK		
GF yogurt (6 oz, nonfat, any flavor)	90	
Coffee or tea	10	100 Cal
LUNCH		
Ham (2 oz) with mustard on 2 slices GF bread	290	
Fresh fruit in season (pear, plum, etc)	70	
Coffee or tea	10	370 Cal
SNACK		
GF Popcorn - Mini Bag (page 85)	100	
Coffee or tea	10	110 Cal
DINNER		
Frozen dinner (Appendix C - page 88)	250	
"Big-Bowl Salad"	150	
GF bread (1 slice)	70	
Water with lemon wedge	10	480 Cal
SNACK		
GF cookie (page 83)	90	
Coffee or tea	10	100 Cal
		1505 Cal

DAY 10 – 1500 Calorie Diet

BREAKFAST	Calories	Totals
Grapefruit (½)	75	
Soft-boiled egg (1)	80	
GF bread - toasted (2 slices)	140	
Coffee	10	305 Cal
SNACK		
GF yogurt (6 oz, nonfat, any flavor)	90	
Coffee or tea	10	100 Cal
LUNCH		
Soup (Appendix D - page 89)	180	
GF bread (1 slice)	70	
Fresh fruit in season (apple, plum, etc)	70	
Coffee or tea	10	330 Cal
SNACK		
GF cookie	60	
Coffee or tea	10	70 Cal
DINNER		
Frozen dinner (Appendix C - page 88)	350	
"Big-Bowl Salad"	150	
Water with lemon wedge	10	580 Cal
SNACK		
Skinny Cow Low Fat Ice Cream Bar (any flavor)	100	
Coffee or tea	10	110 Cal
		1495 Cal

Day 11 – 1500 Calorie Diet

BREAKFAST	Calories	Totals
Grapefruit (½)	75	
Rice Chex (1 cup) + ½ cup skim milk + banana	245	
GF bread - toasted (1 slice)	70	
Coffee	10	400 Cal
SNACK		
Handful unsalted mixed nuts	100	
Coffee or tea	10	110 Cal
LUNCH		
GF Cottage cheese (1 cup no fat)	140	
Fresh fruit in season (apple, peach, plum, etc)	70	
GF bread (1 slice)	70	
Hot or iced tea	10	290 Cal
SNACK		
GF Popcorn - Mini Bag	100	
Coffee or tea	10	110 Cal
DINNER		
Frozen dinner (Appendix C - page 88)	240	
"Big-Bowl Salad"	150	
GF bread (1 slice)	70	
Water with lemon wedge	10	470 Cal
SNACK		
GF cookie (page 83)	90	
Coffee or tea	10	100 Cal
		1480 Cal

DAY 12 – 1500 Calorie

BREAKFAST	Calories	Totals
Orange juice (½ cup)	50	
Scrambled eggs (2)	160	
GF bread - toasted (2 slices)	140	
Coffee	10	360 Cal
SNACK		
GF yogurt (6 oz, nonfat, any flavor) (page 85)	90	
Coffee or tea	10	100 Cal
LUNCH		
Soup (Appendix D - page 89)	160	
Fresh fruit in season (apple, peach, etc)	70	
Coffee or tea	10	240 Cal
SNACK		
GF Popcorn - Mini Bag	100	
Coffee or tea	10	110 Cal
DINNER		
Frozen dinner (Appendix C - page 88)	370	
"Big-Bowl Salad"	150	
GF bread (1 slice)	70	
Water	0	590 Cal
SNACK		
GF cookie (page 83)	90	
Coffee or tea	10	100 Cal
		1510 Cal

DAY 13 – 1500 Calorie

BREAKFAST	Calories	Totals
Orange juice (½ cup)	50	
Rice Krispies* (1 cup) + ½ cup milk + 1 Tbsp raisins	200	
Coffee	10	260 Cal
* Gluten-free variety		
SNACK		
Handful unsalted mixed nuts (page 85)	100	
Coffee or tea	10	110 Cal
LUNCH		
Peanut butter* (2 Tbsp) on 2 slices GF bread	330	
Skim milk (6 oz)	70	
Fresh fruit in season (peach, plum, etc)	70	
Water with lemon wedge	10	480 Cal
* See page 85.		
SNACK		
GF Popcorn - Mini Bag	100	
Coffee or tea	10	110 Cal
DINNER		
Frozen dinner (Appendix C - page 88)	200	
"Big-Bowl Salad"	150	
GF cookie	60	
Coffee or tea	10	420 Cal
SNACK		
Skinny Cow Low Fat Ice Cream Bar (any flavor)	100	
Coffee or tea	10	110 Cal
		1490 Cal

DAY 14 – 1500 Calorie

BREAKFAST	Calories	Totals
Cantaloupe (½ medium)	50	
Oatmeal* (½ cup dry) + ½ cup milk + 1 Tbsp raisins	230	
Coffee	10	290 Cal
* See page 81.		
SNACK		
Fresh fruit in season (apple, peach, etc)	70	
Coffee or tea	10	80 Cal
LUNCH		
Udi's Margherita Pizza*	300	
Diet soda or water	0	300 Cal
* Leftover pizza from Day 7		
SNACK		
Handful unsalted mixed nuts	100	
Coffee or tea	10	110 Cal
DINNER		
Eat Out – Chicken dinner*		
Max allowable calories	610	610 Cal
* See page 11 for eating out tips.		
SNACK		
GF Popcorn - Mini Bag	100	
Coffee or tea	10	110 Cal
		1500 Cal

DAY 15 – 1500 Calorie

BREAKFAST	Calories	Totals
Fresh sliced orange	75	
Cinnamon Chex (¾ cup) + ½ cup milk* + banana	265	
GF bread - toasted (1 slice)	70	
Coffee	10	415 Cal
* Always use skim milk.		
SNACK		
Handful unsalted mixed nuts	100	
Coffee or tea	10	110 Cal
LUNCH		
Soup (Appendix D - page 89)	90	
GF bread (1 slice)	70	
Fresh fruit in season (apple, plum, etc)	70	
Coffee or tea	10	240 Cal
SNACK		
GF Popcorn - Mini Bag	100	
Coffee or tea	10	110 Cal
DINNER		
Frozen dinner (Appendix C - page 88)	320	
"Big-Bowl Salad"	150	
Water with lemon wedge	10	480 Cal
SNACK		
GF cookie (2 cookies)	130	
Coffee or tea	10	140 Cal
		1495 Cal

Day 16 – 1500 Calorie

BREAKFAST	Calories	Totals
Cantaloupe (½ medium)	50	
Rice Chex (1 cup) + ½ cup skim milk + banana	245	
Coffee	10	305 Cal
SNACK		
Handful unsalted mixed nuts	100	
Coffee or tea	10	110 Cal
LUNCH		
Soup (Appendix D - page 89)	100	
GF bread (1 slice)	70	
Fresh fruit in season (pear, plum, etc)	70	
GF Ginger-Snap cookie (page 83)	40	
Coffee or tea	10	290 Cal
SNACK		
GF Popcorn - Mini Bag	100	
Coffee or tea	10	110 Cal
DINNER		
Frozen dinner (Appendix C - page 88)	240	
GF bread (1 slice)	70	
"Big-Bowl Salad"	150	
Coffee or tea	10	470 Cal
SNACK		
Raw Revolution Peanut Butter Chocolate Bar*	200	
Coffee or tea	10	210 Cal
* See page 83.		1495 Cal

DAY 17 – 1500 Calorie

BREAKFAST	Calories	Totals
Orange juice (½ cup)	50	
Fried egg	80	
GF Turkey bacon (3 slices)	105	
GF raisin bread - toasted (2 slices)	140	
Coffee	10	385 Cal
SNACK		
GF yogurt (6 oz, nonfat, any flavor)	90	
Coffee or tea	10	100 Cal
LUNCH		
Soup (Appendix D - page 89)	160	
GF bread (1 slice)	70	
Fresh fruit in season (apple, plum, etc)	70	
Coffee or tea	10	310 Cal
SNACK		
Handful unsalted mixed nuts	100	
Coffee or tea	10	110 Cal
DINNER		
Frozen dinner (Appendix C - page 88)	280	
"Big-Bowl Salad"	150	
Water with lemon wedge	10	440 Cal
SNACK		
GF cookie (2 cookies) (page 83)	130	
Coffee or tea	10	140 Cal
		1485 Cal

DAY 18 – 1500 Calorie

BREAKFAST	Calories	Totals
Grapefruit (½)	75	
Rice Krispies* (1 cup) + ½ cup + 1 Tbsp raisins	200	
GF bread - toasted (1 slice)	70	
Coffee	10	355 Cal
* Gluten-free variety		
SNACK		
Handful unsalted mixed nuts	100	100 Cal
LUNCH		
Cottage cheese (1 cup no fat) (page 85)	140	
Fresh fruit in season (apple, plum, etc)	70	
GF Bread (1 slice)	70	
Water	0	280 Cal
SNACK		
GF Popcorn - Mini Bag	100	100 Cal
DINNER		
Frozen dinner (Appendix C - page 88)	310	
"Big-Bowl Salad"	150	
GF bread (1 slice)	70	
Water	0	530 Cal
SNACK		
GF cookie (2 cookies)	130	
Coffee or tea	10	140 Cal
		1505 Cal

DAY 19 – 1500 Calorie

BREAKFAST	Calories	Totals
Grapefruit (½)	75	
Scrambled egg	80	
GF bread - toasted (2 slices)	140	
Coffee	10	305 Cal
SNACK		
GF yogurt (6 oz, nonfat, any flavor)	90	90 Cal
LUNCH		
Soup (Appendix D - page 89)	200	
GF bread (1 slice)	70	
Fresh fruit in season (peach, plum, etc)	70	
Water with lemon wedge	10	350 Cal
SNACK		
Handful unsalted mixed nuts	100	
Coffee or tea	10	110 Cal
DINNER		
Frozen dinner (Appendix C - page 88)	350	
"Big-Bowl Salad"	150	
GF Ginger-Snap cookie	40	
Coffee or tea	0	570 Cal
SNACK		
GF Popcorn - Mini Bag	100	
Coffee or tea	10	110 Cal
		1505 Cal

DAY 20 – 1500 Calorie

BREAKFAST	Calories	Totals
Fresh or frozen strawberries (½ cup)	25	
Van's Waffles (2) - original or blueberry (page 81)	210	
GF Turkey Breakfast Sausage Links (2)	50	
Light Pancake Syrup* (2 Tbsp) (page 87)	50	
Coffee	10	345 Cal
SNACK		
GF yogurt (6 oz, nonfat, any flavor)	90	
Coffee or tea	10	100 Cal
LUNCH		
Soup (Appendix D - page 89)	160	
GF bread (1 slice)	70	
Fresh fruit in season (apple, peach, etc)	70	
Coffee or tea	10	310 Cal
SNACK		
Handful unsalted mixed nuts (page 85)	100	
Coffee or tea	10	110 Cal
DINNER		
Frozen dinner (Appendix C - page 88)	290	
"Big-Bowl Salad"	150	
GF bread (1 slice)	70	
Water	0	510 Cal
SNACK		
GF Popcorn - Mini Bag (page 85)	100	
Coffee or tea	10	110 Cal
		1485 Cal

Day 21 – 1500 Calorie

BREAKFAST	Calories	Totals
Cantaloupe (½ medium)	50	
Oatmeal (½ cup dry) + ½ cup milk + 1 Tbsp raisins	230	
Coffee	10	290 Cal
SNACK		
Fresh fruit in season (pear, plum, etc)	70	
Coffee or tea	10	80 Cal
LUNCH		
Salad (3 oz canned tuna, 1 tsp Evoo, onions, celery)	175	
Lettuce & tomato wedges	20	
GF bread (1 slice)	70	
Diet soda or water	0	265 Cal
SNACK		
GF Popcorn - Mini Bag (page 85)	100	
Coffee or tea	10	110 Cal
DINNER		
Eat Out – Chicken dinner		
Max allowable calories	650	650 Cal
SNACK		
Handful unsalted mixed nuts	100	
Coffee or tea	10	110 Cal
		1505 Cal

DAY 22 – 1500 Calorie

BREAKFAST	Calories	Totals
Cantaloupe (½ medium)	50	
Cinnamon Chex (¾ cup) + ½ cup milk + ½ banana	215	
Coffee	10	310 Cal
SNACK		
Handful unsalted mixed nuts	100	100 Cal
LUNCH		
Soup (Appendix D - page 89)	150	
GF bread (1 slice)	70	
Fresh fruit in season (apple, plum, etc)	70	
Coffee or tea	10	300 Cal
SNACK		
GF Popcorn - Mini Bag	100	100 Cal
DINNER		
Frozen dinner (Appendix C - page 88)	330	
"Big-Bowl Salad"	150	
GF bread (1 slice)	70	
Water	10	550 Cal
SNACK		
GF cookie (2 cookies)	130	
Coffee or tea	10	140 Cal
		1500 Cal

DAY 23 – 1500 Calorie

BREAKFAST	Calories	Totals
Orange juice (½ cup)	50	
Van's Waffles (2) - original or blueberry	210	
GF Turkey Breakfast Sausage Links (2)	50	
Light Pancake Syrup (2 Tbsp)	50	
Coffee	10	370 Cal
SNACK		
GF yogurt (6 oz, nonfat, any flavor)	90	
Coffee or tea	10	100 Cal
LUNCH		
Ham (2 oz) with mustard on 2 slices GF bread	300	
Pickle spear	0	
Fresh fruit in season (pear, plum, etc)	70	
Coffee or tea	10	380 Cal
SNACK		
Coffee or tea	10	10 Cal
DINNER		
Frozen dinner (Appendix C - page 88)	260	
"Big-Bowl Salad"	150	
Water with lemon wedge	10	420 Cal
SNACK		
Raw Revolution Peanut Butter Chocolate Bar	200	
Coffee or tea	10	210 Cal
		1490 Cal

DAY 24 – 1500 Calorie

BREAKFAST	Calories	Totals
Grapefruit (½)	75	
Scrambled eggs (2)	160	
GF bread - toasted (2 slices)	140	
Coffee	10	385 Cal
SNACK		
GF yogurt (6 oz, nonfat, any flavor)	90	
Coffee or tea	10	100 Cal
LUNCH		
Soup (Appendix D - page 89)	180	
GF bread (1 slice)	70	
Fresh fruit in season (peach, plum, etc)	70	
Coffee or tea	10	330 Cal
SNACK		
GF Popcorn - Mini Bag	100	
Coffee or tea	10	110 Cal
DINNER		
Frozen dinner (Appendix C - page 88)	280	
"Big-Bowl Salad"	150	
Water with lemon wedge	10	440 Cal
SNACK		
GF cookie (2 cookies)	130	
Coffee or tea	10	140 Cal
		1505 Cal

DAY 25 – 1500 Calorie

BREAKFAST	Calories	Totals
Fresh sliced orange	75	
Rice Chex (1 cup) + ½ cup skim milk + banana	245	
GF raisin bread - toasted (1 slice)	70	
Coffee	10	400 Cal
SNACK		
Handful unsalted mixed nuts	100	
Coffee or tea	10	110 Cal
LUNCH		
Cottage cheese (1 cup no fat)	140	
Fresh fruit in season (apple, plum, etc)	70	
GF Bread (1 slice)	70	
Hot or ice tea	10	290 Cal
SNACK		
GF Popcorn - Mini Bag	100	100 Cal
DINNER		
Frozen dinner (Appendix C - page 88)	280	
"Big-Bowl Salad"	150	
GF Bread (1 slice)	70	
Water	0	500 Cal
SNACK		
Handful unsalted mixed nuts	100	
Coffee or tea	10	110 Cal
		1510 Cal

Day 26 – 1500 Calorie

BREAKFAST	Calories	Totals
Orange juice (½ cup)	50	
Fried eggs (2)	160	
GF Turkey bacon (2 slices)	70	
GF bread - toasted (2 slices)	140	
Coffee	10	430 Cal
SNACK		
GF yogurt (6 oz, nonfat, any flavor)	90	
Coffee or tea	10	100 Cal
LUNCH		
Soup (Appendix D - page 89)	200	
GF bread (1 slice)	70	
Fresh fruit in season (apple, peach, etc)	70	
Water with lemon wedge	10	350 Cal
SNACK		
Handful unsalted mixed nuts	100	
Coffee or tea	10	110 Cal
DINNER		
Frozen dinner (Appendix C - page 88)	240	
"Big-Bowl Salad"	150	
Water with lemon wedge	10	400 Cal
SNACK		
Skinny Cow Low Fat Bar (any flavor)	100	
Coffee or tea	10	110 Cal
		1500 Cal

DAY 27 – 1500 Calorie

BREAKFAST	Calories	Totals
Cantaloupe (½ medium)	**50**	
Oatmeal (½ cup dry) + ½ cup milk + 1 Tbsp raisins	**220**	
GF bread - toasted (1 slice)	**70**	
Coffee	**10**	**350 Cal**
SNACK		
Coffee or tea	**10**	**10 Cal**
LUNCH		
Peanut butter (2 Tbsp) on 2 slices GF bread	**330**	
Skim milk (4 oz)	**45**	
Fresh fruit in season (apple, plum, etc)	**70**	
Water	**0**	**445 Cal**
SNACK		
Coffee or tea	**10**	**10 Cal**
DINNER		
Frozen dinner (Appendix C - page 88)	**310**	
"Big-Bowl Salad"	**150**	
Water with lemon wedge	**10**	**470 Cal**
SNACK		
Raw Revolution Peanut Butter Chocolate Bar	**200**	
Coffee or tea	**10**	**210 Cal**
		1495 Cal

DAY 28 – 1500 Calorie

BREAKFAST	Calories	Totals
Orange juice (½ cup)	50	
Rice Krispies* (1 cup) + ½ cup milk + banana	255	
Coffee	10	315 Cal
* Gluten-free variety		
SNACK		
Fresh fruit in season (peach, plum, etc)	70	
Coffee or tea	10	80 Cal
LUNCH		
Salad (3 oz canned tuna, 1 tsp Evoo, onions, celery)	175	
Lettuce & tomato wedges	20	
GF bread (1 slice)	70	
Coffee or tea	10	275 Cal
SNACK		
GF Popcorn - Mini Bag	100	
Coffee or tea	10	110 Cal
DINNER		
Eat Out – Chicken dinner*		
Max allowable calories	610	610 Cal
* See page 11 for eating out tips.		
SNACK		
Skinny Cow Low Fat Bar (any flavor)	100	
Coffee or tea	10	110 Cal
		1500 Cal

DAY 29 – 1500 Calorie

BREAKFAST	Calories	Totals
Grapefruit (½)	75	
Rice Chex (1 cup) + ½ cup skim milk + banana	245	
GF bread - toasted (1 slice)	70	
Coffee	10	400 Cal
SNACK		
Handful unsalted mixed nuts	100	
Coffee or tea	10	110 Cal
LUNCH		
Soup (Appendix D - page 89)	160	
GF bread (1 slice)	70	
Coffee or tea	10	240 Cal
SNACK		
GF Popcorn - Mini Bag	100	
Coffee or tea	10	110 Cal
DINNER		
Frozen dinner (Appendix C - page 88)	270	
"Big-Bowl Salad"	150	
Fresh fruit in season (pear, plum, etc)	70	
Water with lemon wedge	10	500 Cal
SNACK		
GF cookie (2 cookies)	130	
Coffee or tea	10	140 Cal
		1500 Cal

DAY 30 – 1500 Calorie

BREAKFAST	Calories	Totals
Grapefruit (½)	75	
Van's Waffles (2) - original or blueberry	210	
GF Turkey Breakfast Sausage Links (2)	50	
Light Pancake Syrup (2 Tbsp)	50	
Coffee	10	395 Cal
SNACK		
GF yogurt (6 oz, nonfat, any flavor)	90	
Coffee or tea	10	100 Cal
LUNCH		
Ham (2 oz) with mustard on 2 slices GF bread	290	
Fresh fruit in season (apple, plum, etc)	70	
Coffee or tea	10	370 Cal
SNACK		
GF Popcorn - Mini Bag	100	100 Cal
DINNER		
Frozen dinner (Appendix C - page 88)	270	
"Big-Bowl Salad"	150	
Water with lemon wedge	10	430 Cal
SNACK		
Skinny Cow Low Fat Bar (any flavor)	100	
Coffee or tea	10	110 Cal
		1505 Cal

Appendix A
Gluten Notes

Celiac Disease: The primary reason for a gluten-free diet is to combat celiac disease which is a chronic, systemic, autoimmune disorder that causes intestinal damage. Common celiac symptoms include diarrhea, abdominal pain, weight loss and fatigue. On the other hand, some celiac suffers experience constipation instead of diarrhea, weight gain instead of weight loss and heartburn instead of stomach pain. And a few people diagnosed with celiac disease have almost no symptoms. In net, celiac affects many body systems in different ways and because every person displays celiac disease differently, it is a difficult condition to diagnose. A strict gluten-free diet most often alleviates celiac-related symptoms. Keep in mind that all of these possible celiac disease symptoms can be caused by other medical problems. If you suspect you have celiac disease, make sure to see a physician.

Non Celiac Gluten Sensitivity: Another reason to go gluten free is to combat a condition called non-celiac gluten sensitivity that can also affect nearly every system in the body with symptoms that include digestive complaints, skin problems, brain fog, joint pain and numbness in extremities. Because research into this condition is in its early stages, not all physicians have accepted it as an illness and as a result not all physicians provide patients with a diagnosis of gluten sensitivity. Nevertheless, if you believe you suffer from gluten sensitivity, see a physician. To make matters even more confusing, some people are allergic to wheat. These people experience typical allergy symptoms (nasal congestion, etc) and sometimes they also have gastrointestinal symptoms.

Healthier Way to Lose Weight: A new reason to go gluten free is that some medical practitioners believe it is a healthier way to lose weight. But gluten-free weight loss is a recent concept and to date there has not been any research that confirms going gluten free promotes weight loss. Many physicians, however, report a considerable number of their patients claim that when they went gluten free they lost weight and felt a lot better.

Gluten Restriction Levels: Because people with celiac disease and gluten sensitivity have remarkably varying degrees of reaction to trace levels of gluten, it is useful to think in terms of three levels of gluten restriction:

The <u>first level</u> consists of adults with celiac disease. These individuals have a medical reason for being on a gluten-free diet and have serious reactions to gluten. They should avoid not only obvious gluten-laden foods, but also should avoid processed foods that have trace amounts of gluten as well as gluten-free foods that have been cross-contaminated by gluten foods or by trace gluten. (The obvious gluten-laden foods include bread, cereals, and all products with wheat, barley or rye as an ingredient.)

The second level of gluten restriction consists of individuals with non-celiac gluten sensitivity or a wheat allergy who may or may not have a reaction to trace gluten in their food. These people should avoid the obvious gluten containing foods and by trial and error learn what supposedly gluten-free foods (that nevertheless might contain trace gluten) they should also avoid.

In the third level are those who only want to lose weight and feel better on a gluten free diet. These people have only to avoid obvious gluten-containing foods.

Eating Gluten Free in Brief: First, you should be aware of food label ingredients that mean that gluten grains are present: these are triticum vulgare (wheat), triticum spelta (a form of wheat), triticale (cross between wheat and rye), hordeum vulgare (barley) and secale cereale (rye).

Any of the following ingredients on a label indicate that the food definitely contains gluten: wheat protein, hydrolyzed wheat protein, wheat starch, hydrolyzed wheat starch, wheat flour, bread flour, bleached flour, bulgur (a form of wheat), malt (made from barley), couscous (made from wheat), farina (made from wheat), pasta (made from wheat unless otherwise indicated), seitan (made from wheat gluten and commonly found in vegetarian meals) and wheat germ oil or extract (likely cross contaminated).

Any of the following on a label indicate that the food might contain gluten: vegetable protein, hydrolyzed vegetable protein (could be from wheat, corn or soy), modified starch, modified food starch (can come from several sources, including wheat), natural flavor (can be made from barley), artificial flavor (can come from barley), modified food starch, hydrolyzed plant protein (HPP), hydrolyzed vegetable protein (HVP), seasonings, flavorings, vegetable starch, dextrin (sometimes made from wheat) and maltodextrin (sometimes made from wheat).

If a product contains wheat, the FDA requires that it be stated on the food's label. But other gluten-containing grains (barley or rye) do not have to be declared although they might have been added to a food's ingredients. If in doubt, check with the food manufacturer to determine if a food is truly gluten free. (Incidentally, when you call a manufacturer, it is not unusual for them to offer discount coupons for their products!)

Gluten Cross Contamination: Of course, a food that has no gluten-containing ingredients could be cross contaminated with gluten. For example, soybeans and oats do not naturally contain gluten. But soybeans and oats are frequently grown in rotation with wheat crops. That means farmers often use the same fields to grow soy, oats and wheat, they use the same combines to harvest the crops, the same storage facilities and the same trucks to transport the crops to market. As a result, soy and oats are often gluten cross-contaminated.

So if you react to a food that is not supposed to have any gluten ingredients, it is probably because the food contains trace gluten due to cross contamination. The food might have just enough trace gluten to give you problems, despite having an apparently safe list of ingredients.

Appreciate that reactions to gluten vary from person to person. And a gluten reaction is influenced not only by how much gluten is in a food, but also by how much of that food you eat.

Gluten-Free Labeling Standards: The quantity of gluten in a particular product is expressed as parts of gluten contained in a million parts of the product, stated as parts per million, or ppm of gluten. In 2013, the U.S. Food and Drug Administration allowed food manufacturers to label products "gluten-free" that contain less than 20 ppm of gluten (GF 20). Canada the UK and most European Union countries also consider 20 ppm to be gluten free. (20 ppm means a product contains 0.002% gluten). Some people, however, still react to products labeled "gluten-free" that contain less than 20 ppm of gluten. Because of this, several food manufacturers maintain more rigorous standards, typically lowering the amount of gluten in a product to less than 5 or 10 ppm.

Appendix B
Gluten-Free Foods

Because food ingredients and formulations can change at any time, the following lists and recommendations should only be used as a guide. Read the food label and ingredient statement on the food package carefully at the time of purchase to ensure it is gluten free. Moreover, recall that only people with celiac disease and those with extreme gluten sensitivity usually need to be concerned with trace gluten.

And keep in mind our gluten-free guideline: "If in doubt, go without." Do not eat a supposedly gluten-free food if there is no ingredient list or if you are not sure whether the ingredients are gluten-free. If you are unsure of the ingredients, call the food manufacturer for more information.

Finally, although the following list is reasonably comprehensive, it does not contain all the gluten-free foods being sold. And more gluten-free products are continually being developed and found on store shelves.

Baking Mixes, etc: Any baking mix you buy should be labeled "gluten-free." Most baking supplies, such as baking soda, sugar and cocoa, are considered gluten-free, but check ingredients to make certain. Davis, Rumford, Bob's Red Mill and Clabber Girl's baking powder are gluten free.
All Purpose Flour: Bob's Red Mill, King Arthur and other mills make gluten-free all-purpose flour.
Corn Meal: Corn meal should be safe but check the label carefully. Bob's Red Mill makes corn meal in gluten-free factory.
Pancake Mix: Bob's Red Mill, King Arthur, Bisquick and others make gluten free pancake mix.
Pizza Dough: Bob's Red Mill and King Arthur also make gluten free pizza dough.

Bread Products: The gluten in wheat, barley and rye consists of two proteins that combine during the baking process to form a substance that provides bread and other baked goods with elasticity and structure. Gluten also helps bread dough rise into a light, airy loaf. Other grains do not have these characteristics, which is why it is difficult to find passable gluten-free bread. These days many supermarkets stock gluten-free bread, but you often can find a better selection online.
Bread: Udi's Whole Grain Bread (65 Calories per slice), Udi's White Sandwich Bread (70 Calories per slice) and Udi's Cinnamon Raisin Bread (70 Calories per slice), as well as many others are gluten free.
Bread Crumbs: Kinnikinnick Panko-Style Bread Crumbs are gluten free.

Chow Mein Noodles: Goldberg's makes GF chow mein noodles. They are sold in Walmart and many supermarkets.
Hamburger Buns: Kinnikinnick's Hamburger Buns (150 Calories), Rudi's Multi-Grain Hamburger Buns (190 Calories) and Udi's Classic and Whole-Grain Hamburger Buns (190 and 180 Calories per bun) are all gluten free.
Hot Dog Buns: Kinnikinnick's Hot Dog Buns (150 Calories), Rudi's Multi-Grain Hot Dog Buns (140 Calories) and Udi's Classic and Whole-Grain Hot Dog Buns (190 Calories) are all gluten free.
Pita Bread: Toufayan (110 Calories) sells gluten-free wraps.
Polenta: Bob's Red Mill Gluten Free Corn Grits/Polenta is gluten free.

: Some major brands now make several gluten-free cereals:
- General Mills Rice Chex (100 Calories per cup)
- General Mills Corn Chex (120 Calories per cup)
- General Mills Vanilla Chex (120 Calories per ¾ cup)
- General Mills Cinnamon Chex (120 Calories per ¾ cup)
- General Mills Chocolate Chex (130 Calories per ¾ cup)
- General Mills Apple Cinnamon Chex (130 Calories per ¾ cup)
- General Mills Honey Nut Chex (120 Calories per ¾ cup
- Glutino Honey Nut (120 Calories per ¾ cup)
- Glutino Apple Cinnamon (120 Calories per ¾ cup)
- Kellogg's Rice Krispies - gluten-free (110 Calories per cup)
- Cream of Rice (150 Calories per packet)
- Bob's Red Mill Oat Meal
- GF Harvest Oat Meal (150 Calories per cup)
- Waffles: Van's makes six varieties of gluten free waffles.

Coffee, Tea, Soda, Fruit Drinks and Alcohol: Unflavored coffee and black or green tea should be gluten-free, but flavored varieties may not be. Most popular sodas in the United States are gluten-free. Juice that is 100 percent fruit should be gluten-free, but fruit drinks made from fruit plus other ingredients may not be. Conventional beer contains gluten; whereas, wine is gluten-free.

Condiments, Spices & Sauces: In most cases, you will need to check ingredients or call the manufacturer to determine whether their product is gluten free.
BBQ sauces: Sweet Baby Ray's BBQ Sauce (35 Calories per tablespoon any variety), and KC Masterpiece BBQ Sauce (30 Calories per tablespoon any variety) are gluten free.
Cajun Herb-Spice Mix: Cajun's Choice Blackened and Creole Seasoning,

Cajun Quick Shake Seasonings and McCormick's Cajun Seasoning are gluten free.

Herb's & Spices: . Regular salt and pepper should be gluten-free. Fresh herbs and spices in a store's produce section are safe. McCormick's single ingredient spices are gluten-free to 20 parts per million and their spice blends like Italian Seasoning and Salad Supreme Seasoning are gluten free. Check other spice manufacturers for possible gluten cross-contamination.

Marinades: Bone Suckin' Original (also Poultry, Seafood & Steak) Seasoning & Rub and Kikkoman Gluten-Free Teriyaki Marinade & Sauce.

Mustard & Ketchup: French's yellow mustard and Heinz ketchup are gluten-free.

Salsas: The following salsas are gluten free to 20 ppm. All varieties have 5 to 8 Calories per tablespoon.
- Amy's Salsa (mild & medium)
- Amy's Black Bean & Corn
- Farmer's Garden Salsa (medium & hot)
- Farmer's Peach
- Farmer's Pineapple
- Farmer's Roasted Garlic
- Newman's Own Black Bean & Corn
- Ortega Black Bean & Corn
- Ortega Garden Vegetable
- Ortega Original
- Ortega Thick & Chunky
- Ortega Salsa Verde

Soy Sauce: San-J and Kikkoman make gluten-free soy sauce.

Tomato Sauce: The following tomato sauces are both gluten free and low calorie:
- Classico Tomato & Basil Sauce (90 Calories per cup)
- Prego Light Smart Italian Sauce (90 Calories per cup)
- Hunt's Tomato Sauces (80 Calories per cup).

Tomato Paste: Hunt's is gluten free.

Canned Tomatoes: Most canned tomatoes are safe including (but not limited to) Hunt's, Del Monte and Contadina.

Vinegar: Distilled vinegar is derived from gluten grains but usually tests below the 20 ppm gluten threshold and is generally considered safe. Quite a few people with celiac and gluten sensitivity, however, report that they react to both distilled vinegar and distilled alcohol. To be safe, look for cider or balsamic vinegar rather than distilled vinegar.

Worcestershire Sauce: Lea & Perrins and French's Worcestershire Sauce are gluten free. Read the ingredients to make sure nothing has changed.

Cookies & Energy Bars: There are quite a few good tasting gluten-free cookies on the market:
- Glutino's Chocolate Chip cookies, about 60 Calories each
- Glutino's Chocolate Vanilla Creme cookies, about 60 Calories each
- Glutino's Vanilla Creme cookies, about 65 Calories each
- Kinnikinnick's Ginger Snap cookies, about 40 Calories each
- Udi's Chocolate Chip cookies, about 95 Calories each
- Udi's Ginger cookies, about 90 Calories each
- Udi's Oatmeal Raisin cookies, about 90 Calories each
- Udi's Snicker Doodle cookies, about 90 Calories each
Energy Bars: An energy bar is a convenient and sometimes healthy snack. But be careful to choose a brand that comes with protein, vitamins, and minerals, rather than high fructose, corn syrup or sugar. The following are five gluten-free energy bar manufacturers. (There are others.)
- Bumble Bar Organic Energy Bar (about 200 Calories per bar)
- Macrobars Organic Peanut Protein (about 260 Calories)
- NuGo 10 Raw Natural Energy Bar (200 Calories)
- Pure Organic Raw Fruit & Nut Bar (about 200 Calories)
- Raw Revolution Organic Food Bar (about 230 Calories).

Frozen Entrees: Most larger supermarkets have a reasonably good selection of frozen entrees. At this writing, Amy's and Artisan Bistro sell more gluten-free frozen entrees than any other manufacturer. Smart Ones makes two gluten-free entrees. Glutino offers two gluten-free frozen entrees, although each contain 400 Calories. See **Appendix C** (page 88) for a list of Gluten Free frozen entrees available at this writing.

Fruits and Vegetables: Fresh fruits, berries, greens and vegetables are naturally gluten free and generally safe. Most canned fruits and vegetables are gluten-free, but some are not. Single-ingredient frozen fruits and vegetables are generally gluten free, but frozen fruits and vegetables with multiple ingredients frequently contain gluten. Generally, more ingredients in a food increase the chance for trace gluten. Read labels carefully or contact the manufacturer to determine if a particular product is processed in a factory or on manufacturing lines shared with gluten-containing products.

Legumes and Rice: Legumes (lentils, beans, etc) are naturally gluten free, but there is always the risk of cross-contamination during processing and handling. And be wary of canned lentils, beans, etc that have added ingredients. "If in doubt, go without." Brown Rice, white rice, long-grained rice, sticky rice and wild rice are all naturally gluten-free.

Meat, Poultry & Fish: Fresh meat, poultry and fish generally are safe on a gluten-free diet if they are not gluten cross-contaminated at a supermarket or butcher shop. (Realize that the display cases in many stores contain fans that circulate air that could cross-contaminate unprotected meat, poultry and fish. When in doubt choose meat, poultry and fish covered in plastic wrap.)

On the other hand, packaged processed meats, such as hams, bacon, sausages and luncheon meats, could contain gluten. Look for packaged processed meat products labeled gluten-free. Beware of meats and poultry with added ingredients that make them ready-to-cook meals. Most are not safe on a gluten-free diet because the store might have used unsafe ingredients when repackaging the food. Avoid these products.

There are plenty of gluten-free **deli meats**. All of Boar's Head's products are gluten-free and Hormel and Hillshire Farms both make packaged gluten-free meats. But be wary of cross-contamination by shared slicing machines at the deli counter. To make sure deli meat or cheese are gluten free, choose pre-packaged products.

There are lots of **hams** that are considered gluten-free to 20 ppm, although most are not labeled gluten-free. Again check with the manufacturer.

GF **bacon** is widely available. A partial list includes: Applegate Farms, Boar's Head, Jones Dairy Farm, and Wellshire Farms. The following is a partial list of low-calorie gluten-free bacon: Jones Turkey Bacon (35 Calories per slice) and Wellshire Farms Turkey Bacon (40 Calories per slice).

Many **hot dogs** are gluten-free, and a few are labeled gluten-free. A partial list follows: Jennie-O Turkey Franks (95 Calories each), Applegate Chicken Hot Dog (60 Calories each) and Turkey Hot Dog (50 Calories each).

The following is a partial listing of GF **burger patties**: Jennie-O Turkey Burgers (200 Calories each), Applegate Turkey Burgers (140 Calories each) and Beef Burgers (195 Calories each).

GF **veggie burgers** are produced by Amy's, Dr Praeger's and others: Amy's Bistro Veggie Burger (110 Calories) and Sonoma Veggie Burger (140 Calories) and Dr. Praeger's California Veggie Burger (110 Calories).

Many **sausages** contain bread crumbs as a filler, so check labels carefully before buying. In addition, even if the sausage does not include a gluten ingredient, it may have been manufactured on equipment that also processes gluten-containing sausage. The following is a partial list of GF sausage manufacturers: Al Fresco, Applegate Farms, Jones Dairy Farm, Smithfield and Wellshire Farms. Most also produce lower calorie chicken or turkey sausage. (We just tested an Al Fresco chicken sausage, and found it to be tasty, gluten-free and sold in many supermarkets.)

Canned **tuna and salmon** produced by Chicken of the Sea and by Bubble Bee are gluten free.

Milk and Dairy Products: Most milk and many dairy-based products are gluten-free.
Plain, unflavored milk, butter, plain yogurt, fresh eggs and many cheeses are gluten-free. Some ice creams are gluten-free. And many flavored yogurts are gluten-free. Check the ingredients to be sure.
Milk Substitutes: Soy, rice and almond milk are most often gluten-free, but some are not. Check the labels. (Soy, rice and almond milk may be substituted for cow's skim milk provided the calorie count is close.)
Yogurt: All varieties of Chobani and Yoplait yogurt, including flavored varieties, are gluten free. Yoplait Light in the 6 oz container has 90 Calories.
Cheeses: Most cheeses are naturally gluten-free. One slice (1 oz) of light cheese has about 70 Calories. Beware of cheese that has been sliced and repackaged at a supermarket. It might be cross contaminated. Usually, it is safer to buy cheese that has been packaged at the manufacturer's plant.
Cottage Cheese: Breakstone, Cabot, Humboldt and others make fat free, gluten-free cottage cheese.
Ice Cream: Although many ice cream products are gluten free, some are not. Also consider GF frozen fruit pops. All of Skinny Cow's ice cream bars are gluten free: Chocolate Truffle Bar (100 Calories), Caramel Truffle Bar (100 Calories) and Fudge Bars (110 Calories).

Oils, Nuts & Popcorn: Most oils (olive, canola, etc), nuts, and popcorn varieties are gluten free. Nuts are naturally gluten free. But beware of nuts and popcorn with added flavorings that might contain gluten. Some popcorn brands that are considered gluten free are Jolly Time, Newman's Own and Orville Redenbacher's.
Peanut Butter: Arrowhead Mills and Smart Balance peanut butter are gluten free (about 95 Calories per tablespoon.)
Mayonnaise: Hellmann's and Best Foods regular and light mayonnaise are gluten free. (light is 35 Calories per serving)
Non-Stick Cooking Spray: Original Pam, Mazola and Wegman's store brand cooking sprays are gluten free.

Pasta: Fortunately, there are a number of gluten-free pastas available, in different shapes and sizes. Choose gluten-free pasta made from rice or corn rather than wheat. Surprisingly, many of these gluten-free varieties are quite good, making it possible to serve gluten-free pasta whose taste is very close to wheat-based pasta. The following manufacturers make gluten-free pasta: Ancient Harvest, Andean Dream, Bionaturae, Jovial, DeBoles, DeLallo, Le Veneziane, Lundberg, Riso Bello, Rizopia, Ronzoni, Rustichella D'Abruzzo, Sam Mills and Tinkyada.

Salad Dressings: When buying vinaigrette-type salad dressings look for cider or balsamic vinegar, not distilled vinegar on the food label. (Distilled vinegar is made from gluten grains.) The following salad dressings are gluten free:
- Annie's Lite Raspberry Vinaigrette (20 Calories per tablespoon)
- Annie's Lite Italian Dressing (23 Calories per tablespoon)
- Annie's Lite Honey Mustard Vinaigrette (20 Calories per tablespoon)
- Annie's Lite Herb Balsamic Vinaigrette (25 Calories per tablespoon)
- Annie's Lite Gingerly Vinaigrette (20 Calories per tablespoon).
- Gazebo Room Lite Greek Salad Dressing (20 Calories per tablespoon)
- Ken's Lite Options Italian w/ Romano & Red Pepper (23 Calorie per tablespoon)
- Newman's Own Lite Balsamic Vinaigrette (13 Calorie per tablespoon)
- Newman's Own Lite Roasted Garlic Balsamic (25 Calories per tablespoon)
- Newman's Own Lite Red Wine Vinaigrette & Olive Oil (25 Calories per tablespoon)
- Newman's Own Lite Low-Fat Sesame Ginger (18 Calories per tablespoon)
- San-J's Tamari Sesame Salad Dressing (20 Calories per tablespoon)
- San-J's Tamari Ginger Salad Dressing (13 Calories per tablespoon)
- Sophia's Oil-Free Cilantro & Lime (5 Calories per tablespoon)

Soups (See **Appendix D**, page 91 for a list of GF soup.)
<u>Amy's Kitchen</u>: A great many of Amy's 29 soups are considered gluten-free to 20 ppm.
<u>Bookbinders Specialties</u>: This gourmet soup company has 11 gluten-free soups. All are tested to below 20 ppm, and are available by mail order or in U.S. supermarkets in the northeast.
<u>Frontier Soup</u>: Frontier makes 28 varieties of gluten-free soup mixes. All are certified to below 5ppm of gluten. Frontier Soup mixes are available online and at upscale supermarket chains.
<u>Imagine Foods</u>: Imagine Foods claims all varieties of its soups are gluten-free to 20 ppm except for Organic Creamy Chicken and Imagine Bistro Bisques. Imagine soups are usually found in the "natural foods" section of supermarkets.
<u>Pacific Foods</u>: Almost all Pacific's soups are gluten free. Most often Pacific soups are found in the natural or health food section of a supermarket,

although in some stores they are next to conventional soups.

<u>Progresso</u>: Choose from Progresso's many gluten-fee varieties tested to 20 ppm.

Stock, Broth & Bouillon: Stock is made by simmering vegetables, bones, meat scraps, etc, and is the best base for soups, stews, and sauces. Unfortunately stock is rarely found on supermarket shelves. Broth is stock with added salt and can be used in the same way as homemade stock -- although broth is not as rich and complex as stock. Bouillon is dehydrated stock formed into cubes or granules. It is convenient but is typically processed with large amounts of sodium and other additives. Thus the liquid it produces is almost flavorless.

Kitchen Basics makes gluten free Chicken, Beef, Vegetable, Turkey, Seafood, Veal, Unsalted Chicken and Unsalted Beef stock. Pacific Foods sells gluten free vegetable broth, mushroom broth, beef broth and chicken and vegetable stock. College Inn's garden-vegetable broth, organic-beef broth, tender-beef bold stock and white wine & herb broth are all considered gluten-free to 20ppm. Hormel's vegetable, beef and chicken bouillon cubes are gluten free.

Miscellaneous

We put food products in this category that did not seem to fit anywhere else.

<u>Pancake Syrup</u>: Hungry Jack Lite Syrup (25 Calories per tablespoon), Log Cabin Lite Syrup (25 Calories per tablespoon) and Vermont Maid Lite Syrup (30 Calories per tablespoon) are gluten free.

Appendix C
Frozen Entrees

Amy's GF Frozen Entrees (12)
- Amy's Quinoa, Black Beans, Butternut Squash & Chard (**240 Cal**)
- Amy's Black Bean & Cheese Enchilada (**240 Cal**)
- Amy's Mushroom Risotto Bowl (**240 Cal**)
- Amy's Sweet & Sour Asian Noodle Bowl (**250 Cal**)
- Amy's Vegetable Parmesan Bowl (**260 Cal**)
- Amy's Brown Rice & Veggies Bowl – Light Sodium (**260 Cal**)
- Amy's Brown Rice, Black-eyed Peas & Veggies Bowl (**290 Cal**)
- Amy's Teriyaki Bowl (**290 Cal**)
- Amy's Asian Noodle Stir Fry (**300 Cal**)
- Amy's Vegetable Lasagna (**300 Cal**)
- Amy's Thai Stir-Fry (**310 Cal**)
- Amy's Tofu Scramble (**320 Cal**)

Artisan Bistro GF Frozen Entrees (18)
- Artisan Bistro Wild Alaskan Salmon (**200 Cal**)
- Artisan Bistro Chicken Parmesan Bake (**200 Cal**)
- Artisan Bistro Turkey Cheddar Bake (**240 Cal**)
- Artisan Bistro Wild Alaskan Salmon Bake (**240 Cal**)
- Artisan Bistro Thai Style Yellow Curry with Chicken (**240 Cal**)
- Artisan Bistro Cheddar Beef Bake (**250 Cal**)
- Artisan Bistro Sesame Ginger with Salmon (**270 Cal**)
- Artisan Bistro Coconut Lemongrass with Chicken (**270 Cal**)
- Artisan Bistro Spiced Chicken Morocco (**270 Cal**)
- Artisan Bistro Albacore Tuna Bake (**280 Cal**)
- Artisan Bistro Thai Style Red Curry with Beef (**280 Cal**)
- Artisan Bistro Chicken Citron (**280 Cal**)
- Artisan Bistro Wild Alaskan Salmon with Pesto (**310 Cal**)
- Artisan Bistro Savory Turkey (**330 Cal**)
- Artisan Bistro Southwest Style Beef (**330 Cal**)
- Artisan Bistro Ginger Chicken (**350 Cal**)
- Artisan Bistro Beef with Mushroom Sauce (**350 Cal**)
- Artisan Bistro Wild Alaskan Salmon Cake (**370 Cal**)

Smart Ones GF Frozen Entrees (2)
- Smart Ones Lemon Herb Chicken Piccata (**250 Cal**)
- Smart Ones Santa Fe Style Rice & Beans (**290 Cal**)

Appendix D
Gluten-Free Soup

Soup Description	Calories*
Amy's Vegetable Barley Soup	70
Progresso Chicken Rice with Vegetables Soup	80
Amy's Alphabet Soup	80
Pacific Chicken Noodle Soup	90
Progresso Vegetable Classics Garden Vegetable Soup	90
Amy's Split Pea Soup	100
Pacific Butternut Squash Bisque	110
Amy's Cream of Tomato Soup	110
Progresso Traditional Manhattan Clam Chowder	110
Pacific Roasted Red Pepper & Tomato Soup	110
Amy's Mushroom Bisque with Porcini	120
Amy's Pasta & 3 Bean Soup	130
Pacific Chicken Spinach Penne Soup	140
Amy's Hearty Minestrone with Vegetables Soup	150
Amy's Summer Corn & Vegetable Soup	150
Progresso Vegetable Classics Lentil Soup	160
Amy's Tuscan Bean & Rice Soup	160
Progresso Hearty New England Clam Chowder	180
Progresso Potato Broccoli & Cheese Chowder	200

* Calories per serving. When the Daily Meal Plan menu specifies soup, have only one serving (8 ounces) unless stated otherwise. (Note cans of soup usually contain about two servings.) See page 86 for additional gluten-free soup manufacturers.

Appendix E
Exercise Smart

Our bodies are just not built to be immobile and passive. The sad fact, however, is that after years of education and information programs by government agencies, medical associations and insurance companies, relatively few Americans engage in regular
planned exercise – despite the reality that we need to be active to keep our systems working efficiently and rid ourselves of emotional tension. Moreover, exercise burns calories, speeds up your metabolism and is an invaluable part of any weight control program. There are two ways to become more physically active: 1) Increase the physical activity in your daily life; and 2) Start on a regular exercise program. Better still would be a combination of both. Simply stated, there are three basic types of exercise: aerobic, stretching and strengthening.

Aerobic Exercises (also called "cardio") condition your cardiovascular system. Aerobic exercises, such as jogging, swimming, cycling, brisk walking, skipping rope, and many others, are typically deep breathing and continuous, with rhythmic and repetitive contractions of your large muscle groups. The trait most aerobic exercises have in common is that they make you work hard and require you process a great deal of oxygen.

Some typical aerobic exercises are: Most strenuous include bicycling, cross-country skiing, dancing (aerobic), hiking in rugged terrain, ice hockey, jogging, jogging in place, rowing, skipping rope, stair climbing, and stationary cycling. Somewhat less strenuous are basketball, field hockey, calisthenics, handball, racquetball, skiing (downhill), soccer, squash, tennis (singles), volleyball, and walking (briskly). Least strenuous aerobic exercises consist of badminton, baseball, bowling, croquet, dancing, gardening, golf (carrying or pulling clubs), horseback riding, housework, ping-pong, shuffleboard, softball, tennis (doubles) and walking (moderate to leisurely).

Stretching-type Exercises such as yoga, tai chi, Pilates and to a lesser extent calisthenics can improve your flexibility – and some of the exercises can make you somewhat stronger.

As you age you inevitably start to loose flexibility. Your gait becomes stiffer; you can't stand quite as upright as you used to; it becomes tougher to bend over; and you have difficulty turning your neck. Regardless of your age, however, stretching can make you more flexible, less injury prone, and can reduce the pain and discomfort associated with tight muscles and shortened tendons. Realize, however, that stretching exercises do not condition your heart and lungs. Stretching exercises are fine as long as they are performed in addition to rather than in place of an aerobic exercise.

Most experts do recommend stretching before and after an aerobic or strength routine. However, never stretch cold muscles and always do some form of warm up prior to stretching. Stretch slowly and hold gently. You should stretch to the point of feeling a mild pull, but you should never feel pain. And when you stretch – do not bounce.

Muscle Building and Strengthening Exercises, e.g., weight lifting, use of the machines found in fitness centers and isometrics.

Once more, as you age you loose muscle mass, your bone density decreases and you lose strength. Exercises like weight lifting strengthen your muscles, bones and joints. Strengthening exercises also reduce your risk of developing osteoporosis, a severe bone-loss disease, which can lead to easily fractured bones and all the complications that often follow. Strong muscles not only allow you to lift a sleepy four-year old out of a car without difficulty and lug groceries up to a second floor apartment, but as with increased flexibility, strong muscles also make you less injury prone. Moreover, because **muscle uses many more calories than fat, when you replace fat with muscle, your metabolism actually speeds up.**

100-Day Super Diet-1200 Calorie*	Weight Loss for Men - Metric*
100-Day Super Diet-1500 Calorie*	Maximum Weight Loss- 1200 Calorie*
100-Day No-Cooking Diet-1200 Cal*	Maximum Weight Loss- 1500 Calorie*
100-Day No-Cooking Diet-1500 Cal*	Weight Control - U.S. Edition
90-Day Smart Diet-1200 Calorie*	Weight Control - Metric. Edition
90-Day Smart Diet-1500 Calorie*	Professional Weight Control Women - U.S.
90-Day No-Cooking Diet - 1200 Cal*	Professional Weight Control Women - Metric
90-Day No-Cooking Diet - 1500 Cal*	Professional Weight Control Men - U.S.
90-Day Perfect Diet - 1200 Calorie*	Professional Weight Control Men - Metric
90-Day Perfect Diet - 1500 Calorie*	Weight Maintenance - U.S. Edition*
60-Day Perfect Diet-1200 Calorie*	Weight Maintenance - Metric. Edition*
60-Day Perfect Diet-1500 Calorie*	Weight Maintenance - UK Edition
50-Day Flex Diet-1200 Calorie*	Weight Loss for Senior Men*
50-Day Flex Diet-1500 Calorie*	Weight Loss for Senior Women*
30-Day Quick Diet - for Women*	Eat Smart - U.S. Edition*
30-Day Quick Diet - for Men*	Eat Smart - Metric Edition
30-Day No-Cooking Diet*	30-Day Mediterranean Diet
30-Day Diet for Women - Metric*	Exercise Smart - U.S. Edition*
30-Day Diet for Men - Metric*	Exercise Smart - Metric Edition
25 Day Easy Diet-1200 Calorie*	Exercise Smart - UK Edition*
25 Day Easy Diet-1500 Calorie*	Total Fitness - U.S. Edition
25-Day No-Cooking Diet	Total Fitness - Metric Edition
10-Day Express Diet	Total Fitness - UK Edition
10-Day No-Cooking Diet*	Total Fitness for Women-U.S. Edition*
7-Day Diet for Women*	Total Fitness for Women - Metric
7-Day Diet for Men*	Total Fitness for Women - UK Edition
7-Day No-Cooking Diets*	Total Fitness for Men - U.S. Edition*
90-Day Gluten-Free Diet-1200 Cal*	Total Fitness for Men- Metric Edition*
90-Day Gluten-Free Diet-1500 Cal*	Total Fitness for Men - UK Edition
30-Day Gluten-Free Quick Diet*	Senior Fitness - U.S. Edition*
30-Day Gluten-Free No-Cooking Diet*	Senior Fitness - Metric Edition*
7-Day Diet for Women - Metric*	Senior Fitness - UK Edition*
7-Day Diet for Men - Metric	Computer Diet - U.S. Edition*
7-Day Gluten-Free Express Diet*	Computer Diet - Metric Edition*
7-Day Gluten-Free No-Cooking Diet*	Reliable Weight Loss - U.S. Edition
90-Day Vegetarian Diet-1200 Calorie*	101 Weight Loss Tips*
90-Day Vegetarian Diet-1500 Calorie*	101 Healthy Eating Tips*
30-Day Vegetarian Diet*	101 Lifelong Fitness Tips*
7-Day Vegetarian Diet*	101 Weight Maintenance Tips
Weight Loss for Women*	101 Weight Loss Recipes
Weight Loss for Women - Metric	101 Gluten-Free Weight Loss Recipes
Weight Loss for Women - UK	101 Vegetarian Weight Loss Recipes*
Weight Loss for Men*	30-Day Mediterranean Diet*
Maximum Weight Loss - 1200 Cal*	90-Day Mediterranean Diet - 1200 Cal*
Maximum Weight Loss - 1500 Cal*	90-Day Mediterranean Diet - 1500 Cal*

* These titles are available as both ebooks and paperbacks. Our ebooks are sold by Amazon, Apple, Google, Barnes & Noble and Kobo. But our paperbacks are only sold by Amazon.

Disclaimer

This book offers general meal planning, nutrition and weight control information. It is not a medical manual and the authors do not claim to be medically qualified. Everyone should have a medical checkup before beginning this gluten-free weight loss program. Moreover, the physician conducting the medical exam should be made aware of and should approve this diet. Because commercial food ingredients and formulations can change at any time, adults with celiac disease or gluten sensitivity should be particularly careful and double check the ingredients in the foods listed in this book to be sure they are gluten free. We recommend that you do not solely rely on the information presented here and that you always read labels, warnings, and directions before using or consuming a product. For additional information about a product, please contact the manufacturer. The content on this site is for reference purposes and is not intended to substitute for advice given by a physician, pharmacist, or other licensed health-care professional. You should not use this information as self-diagnosis or for treating a health problem or disease. Contact your health-care provider immediately if you suspect that you have a medical problem. Additionally, while the authors and publisher have made every effort to ensure the accuracy of the information in this book, they make no representations or warranties regarding its accuracy or completeness. Further, neither the authors nor publisher assume liability for any medical problems that might result from applying the methods in this book, or for any loss of profit, or any other commercial damages, including but not limited to special, incidental, consequential or other damages, and any such liability is hereby expressly disclaimed.